Pediatric Medical Emergencies

What Do I Do Now?: Emergency Medicine

SERIES EDITOR-IN-CHIEF

Catherine A. Marco, MD, FACEP
Professor, Emergency Medicine & Surgery
Wright State University Boonshoft School of Medicine
Dayton, Ohio

Pediatric Medical Emergencies

Edited by

Ann M. Dietrich, MD, FAAP, FACEP
Associate Professor of Pediatrics
Ohio University
Heritage College of Medicine
Medical Director of Education
Ohio ACEP
Columbus, OH

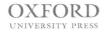

OXFORD
UNIVERSITY PRESS

OXFORD
UNIVERSITY PRESS

Oxford University Press is a department of the University of Oxford. It furthers
the University's objective of excellence in research, scholarship, and education
by publishing worldwide. Oxford is a registered trade mark of Oxford University
Press in the UK and certain other countries.

Published in the United States of America by Oxford University Press
198 Madison Avenue, New York, NY 10016, United States of America.

Library of Congress Cataloging-in-Publication Data
Names: Dietrich, Ann M., editor.
Title: Pediatric medical emergencies / [edited by] Ann M. Dietrich.
Other titles: What do I do now?
Description: New York, NY : Oxford University Press, [2020] |
Series: What do I do now? | Includes bibliographical references and index.
Identifiers: LCCN 2019041109 (print) | LCCN 2019041110 (ebook) |
ISBN 9780190946678 (hb) | ISBN 9780190946692 (epub) |
ISBN 9780190946708 | ISBN 9780190946715
Subjects: MESH: Pediatric Emergency Medicine |
Emergencies | Emergency Treatment | Child | Infant | Adolescent | Case Reports
Classification: LCC RJ370 (print) | LCC RJ370 (ebook) | NLM WS 205 | DDC 618.92/0025—dc23
LC record available at https://lccn.loc.gov/2019041109
LC ebook record available at https://lccn.loc.gov/2019041110

9 8 7 6 5 4 3 2 1

Printed by Marquis, Canada

Contents

Contributors

Nina Ackerman, MD
Emergency Medicine, Long
Island Jewish Medical Center,
Northwell Health
New Hyde Park, NY

Lauren Allister, MD
Pediatric Emergency Medicine,
Hasbro Children's Hospital/Warren
Alpert Medical School of Brown
University
Providence, RI

**Isabel Barata, MS, MD, MBA,
FACP, FAAP, FACEP**
Associate Professor of Pediatrics
and Emergency Medicine, Zucker
School of Medicine at Hofstra/
Northwell; Pediatric Emergency
Medicine Service Line Quality
Director, Emergency Medicine and
Pediatrics Service Line; Director
of Pediatric Emergency Medicine,
North Shore University Hospital
Manhasset, NY

Katherine Battisti, MD
Department of Emergency
Medicine, Nationwide Children's
Hospital
Columbus, OH

Bridget Bonaventura, MD
Pediatric Emergency Medicine,
Nationwide Children's Hospital,
Ohio State University
Columbus, OH

Beth Bubolz, MD
Pediatric Emergency Medicine,
Nationwide Children's Hospital,
Ohio State University
Columbus, OH

Hannah Carter, MD
Department of Emergency
Medicine, Northwell Health—
North Shore University Hospital/
Long Island Jewish Medical
Centers, Donald and Barbara
Zucker School of Medicine at
Hofstra/Northwell
Manhasset, NY

Crista Cerrone, MD
Division of Emergency Medicine,
Nationwide Children's Hospital,
Department of Pediatrics,
The Ohio State University
Columbus, OH

Meghan Dishong, MD
Department of Pediatrics,
Emergency Medicine, Nationwide
Children's Hospital
Columbus, OH

Maytal Firnberg, MD
Department of Emergency
Medicine, Division of Pediatric
Emergency Medicine, Columbia
University Medical Center/Morgan
Stanley Children's Hospital
New York, NY

David Foster, MD
Department of Emergency
Medicine, North Shore University
Hospital
Manhasset, NY

Susana Ho, MD
Emergency Medicine Resident,
PGY2, Northwell Health at North
Shore University Hospital and
Long Island Jewish Hospital
Manhasset, NY

Dana Libov, DO
Resident in Emergency Medicine,
North Shore-Long Island Jewish
Health System/Hofstra North
Shore-Long Island Jewish School
of Medicine at North Shore
University Hospital
Manhasset, NY

**Sharon E. Mace, MD,
FACEP, FAAP**
Professor of Medicine,
Cleveland Clinic Lerner College
of Medicine at Case Western
Reserve University,
Director of Research, Cleveland
Clinic, Associate Director of EMS
Cleveland Clinic Health Systems,
Former Director of Pediatric
Education and Quality
Improvement and Director
Observation Unit,
Cleveland Clinic
Cleveland, OH

Laurie Malia, DO
Department of Emergency
Medicine, Division of Pediatric
Emergency Medicine, Columbia
University Medical Center/Morgan
Stanley Children's Hospital
New York, NY

Melissa A. McGuire, MD
Assistant Professor, Department of
Emergency Medicine, Northwell
Health at North Shore University
Hospital and Cohen Children's
Medical Center
Manhasset, NY

Athena Mihailos, MD, MPH
Director of Emergency Ultrasound,
Long Island Jewish Medical Center,
Assistant Professor, Zucker
School of Medicine at Hofstra/
Northwell, Department of
Emergency Medicine, Long
Island Jewish Medical Center at
Northwell Health
New Hyde Park, NY

Pinaki Mukherji, MD
Department of Emergency
Medicine, Northwell Health Long
Island Jewish Medical Center
New Hyde Park, NY

Nkeiruka Orajiaka, MD, MPH
Department of Pediatrics,
Emergency Medicine, Nationwide
Children's Hospital
Columbus, OH

Christopher Perry, MD
Department of Emergency
Medicine, Long Island Jewish
Medical Center
New Hyde Park, NY

Ajay K. Puri, MD
Resident, Department of
Emergency Medicine, Northwell
Health at North Shore University
Hospital and Long Island Jewish
Medical Center
Manhasset, NY

Renee Quarrie, MBBS, FAAP
Department of Pediatric
Emergency Medicine, University of
Maryland Medical Center
Baltimore, MD

Joni E. Rabiner, MD
Department of Emergency
Medicine, Division of Pediatric
Emergency Medicine, Columbia
University Medical Center/Morgan
Stanley Children's Hospital
New York, NY

Sriram Ramgopal, MD
Department of Pediatrics,
Division of Pediatric Emergency
Medicine, Children's Hospital of
Pittsburgh
Pittsburgh, PA

Trupti Shah, MD, FACEP
Director of Medical Student
Clerkship, Emergency Medicine
Ultrasound,
Assistant Professor, Zucker
School of Medicine at Hofstra/
Northwell, Department of
Emergency Medicine, Long
Island Jewish Medical Center at
Northwell Health
New Hyde Park, NY

Sakina Sojar, MD
Pediatric Emergency Medicine,
Hasbro Children's Hospital/Warren
Alpert Medical School of Brown
University
Providence, RI

Nechama Sonenthal, MD
Department of Emergency
Medicine, Long Island Jewish
Medical Center
New Hyde Park, NY

Michael Sperandeo, MD
Department of Emergency
Medicine, Northwell Health—
North Shore University Hospital/
Long Island Jewish Medical
Centers, Donald and Barbara
Zucker School of Medicine at
Hofstra/Northwell
Manhasset, NY

Michael J. Stoner, MD
Division of Emergency Medicine,
Nationwide Children's Hospital
Department of Pediatrics,
The Ohio State University
Columbus, OH

Richard Tang, MD
Emergency Medicine Resident,
Zucker School of Medicine-
Northwell at North Shore
University Hospital/Long Island
Jewish Medical Center
Hempstead, NY

Tracey Wagner, MD
Department of Emergency
Medicine, Nationwide Children's
Hospital
Columbus, OH

1 No Poop

Michael Sperandeo and Isabel Barata

A 3-day-old male is brought to the emergency
department by the parents with a chief complaint
of fever and abdominal distention. The patient was
born at home under the guidance of a midwife. Since
birth, the parents have noticed decreased ability to
tolerate feedings and increased lethargy. The parents
report the child has not yet passed meconium. The
patient was born full term by vaginal delivery. On
exam, the patient appears ill, lethargic, and minimally
responsive to tactile stimuli and appears warm and
clammy with marked abdominal distention. Vital
signs are: HR 222, SBP 55, RR 55, T 102.4°F (39.1°C),
SpO_2 98% on room air. The patient weighs 2.5 kg (5.5
lbs). On exam you note a distended, firm, tympanic
abdomen. The child is spitting up bilious stained
vomitus. On rectal exam the anal orifice appears
patent; shortly after digital rectal exam the patient
experiences explosive, florid, watery meconium
stained diarrhea. There are no rashes.

What do you do now?

DISCUSSION

A lethargic, ill-appearing neonate with vital signs concerning for septic shock in the setting of a distended abdomen and failure to pass meconium, is an emotionally and medically challenging case presentation for any emergency medicine provider. A neonate with failure to pass meconium within the first 24 to 48 hours should raise the provider's suspicion for Hirschsprung's disease (HD).[1,2] In this case, abnormal vital signs, fever, septic shock, a surgical distended abdomen, and florid diarrhea after digital rectal exam points to one of the more dreaded complications of HD, Hirschsprung-associated enterocolitis (HAEC).[3]

Hirschsprung's disease (congenital megacolon) affects approximately 1 in 5,000 births with a male to female ratio of 4:1. Aganglionosis of the enteric nervous system in the myenteric and submucosal plexuses of the distal intestine characterize HD.[4-6] The resulting lack of peristalsis in the large bowel leads to a functional bowel obstruction. Though the exact etiology of HD is not known, it is believed that incomplete or failure of migration of distal ganglion cells leads to an area of aganglionosis. Normal neural crest ganglionic cells migrate along the gastrointestinal tract during the 5th through 12th weeks of gestation. There is some evidence that not all cases of HD may be secondary to failure of migration but may be to failure of terminal ganglionic cells differentiation.[6] Classically, the aganglionic segment begins at the internal anal sphincter and extends a variable distance proximally. Most are limited to the rectosigmoid area; however, a minority of cases may extend proximally to the splenic flexure. In other rare, most severe cases, an aganglionic segment may involve the entire length of both the large and small intestines.[2,7] Regardless of the length of the aganglionic bowel, the functional obstruction always includes internal anal sphincter dysfunction.[5]

Both the internal and external anal sphincters mediate normal defecation. The internal sphincter is composed of tonically contracted smooth muscle, whereas the external anal sphincter maintains continence via voluntary skeletal muscle contraction and relaxation. When stool fills the rectum, stretch receptors allow for the disinhibition of neuronal cells in the internal anal sphincter, thus allowing for relaxation; thereafter-voluntary external sphincter muscles contract allowing for the expulsion of stool. In HD, this neuronal axis is disrupted and internal sphincter contraction does not relax with bowel distention.[6]

At the macroscopic level, the bowel in HD patients contains a narrow aganglionic segment, a proximal transition zone progressing from a narrow to dilated lumen and a dilated proximal portion of bowel. These findings are often demonstrated on abdominal plain films and on barium contrast enema.[1,4–6]

Most cases of HD occur as isolated phenomena. However, family history has been implicated in 7% of cases and as high as 20% in cases of HD involving longer segments of bowel. Families with a member with HD are at 200 times increased risk of recurrence.[5] In addition, HD is 10 times more frequent in patients with Down syndrome when compared to the general population. Furthermore, 2% of patients with congenital aganglionosis have Down syndrome. Other disorders with an association with HD include Waardenberg syndrome, Smith-Lemli-Opitz syndrome, Laurence-Moon-Biedl-Bardet syndrome, and Haddad syndrome (congenital central hypoventilation).[5–7]

SIGNS, SYMPTOMS, AND DIFFERENTIAL DIAGNOSIS

Most cases of HD are diagnosed in the first 2 days of life with a presentation of bile stained vomit and abdominal distention; however, it may present with intermittent episodes in less severe cases. Constipation and failure to pass meconium is often one of the chief presenting complaints from parents in children with HD. Though there are many causes of constipation, 90% of children with HD will have a reported history of failure to spontaneously pass meconium within the first 48 hours of life. On the other hand, 99% of term and 95% of preterm infants will spontaneously pass meconium by 48 hours.[7,8] In diagnosis outside of the neonatal period, 80% of patients will have a reported history of difficult bowel movements, poor feeding, and progressive abdominal distention. Despite these associations, in children with failure to pass meconium within the first 48 hours, meconium-plug syndrome and cystic fibrosis related meconium ileus are both more prevalent than HD.[8–9] In developing countries or in settings with limited healthcare resources, HD may be initially overlooked. In these cases, older undiagnosed children may present or report a history of persisting and chronic symptoms consistent with partial bowel obstruction. Older children often present thin appearing, with developmental delays and with failure to thrive.[2,5,8] When these children do pass stools, they are often subject to irregular and uncomfortable bowel movements. On physical examination, in addition to noting a potentially firm or distended abdomen, the rectum is often empty on digital rectal exam. If the examiner palpates proximally to the aganglionic segment, an episode of frank, explosive soft stools and diarrhea may occur.[5–7]

When considering diagnostic modalities to evaluate the presence of HD, it is helpful to regard HD as similar to a partial or functional bowel obstruction. As such, radiological findings are typically consistent with what one would expect with a bowel obstruction. An upright abdominal plain film x-ray will often demonstrate abdominal distention with distended loops of bowel, air fluid levels, and absence of rectal air or a narrow rectum. Barium contrast enema will often demonstrate a reduced rectosigmoid section with a thin transition zone to a more distended, proximal colon. The aganglionic segment may also demonstrate a "sawtooth" appearance thought to be secondary to intermittent muscular fasciculation and/or bowel wall edema. Failure to clear contrast is also a reliable sign of HD; in this setting repeat films should be considered. Evaluation of the rectosigmoid ratio (R/S ratio) in patients with more distal disease may be helpful when interpreting imaging studies. The rectosigmoid ratio is the ratio of the diameter of the rectum compared to that of the sigmoid colon with a normal ratio ≥1. Patients with an R/S ratio of less than one suggest a diagnosis of HD.[4,5]

Though radiographic modalities may aid in the diagnosis of HD, definitive diagnosis rests with rectal suction biopsy or full thickness rectal biopsies. The absence of ganglionic cells in the intramuscular myenteric plexus and the submucosal Meissner's plexus remains as the classic histological finding in HD.[4–7]

HIRSCHSPRUNG-ASSOCIATED ENTEROCOLITIS

The most concerning complication of HD is that of HAEC. HAEC is the leading cause of morbidity and mortality and is responsible for nearly half the deaths associated with HD. HAEC can occur both in the preoperative and perioperative periods and, like HD, has a strong association with Down syndrome.[1] Despite the severity of HAEC, there is currently no standard definition of HAEC. Lack of a definitional consensus is likely secondary to both varying definitions by different surgical groups as well as poorly understood pathophysiology.[3] It is currently believed that the etiology and severity of HAEC is multifactorial, likely involving a combination of a dysfunctional enteric nervous system leading to functional bowel obstruction and colitis, insufficient IgA immunoglobulin secretion, increased mucin production, and disruption of the normal intestinal biome.[3,5] Despite these definitional shortcomings, Pastor et al. have developed a scoring system for identifying patients clinically concerning for HAEC. Included in this scoring system are symptoms consistent with HD, necrotizing enterocolitis, and bowel obstruction. Each item is given a value of 1 or 2, with a total score of greater than or equal to 10 as concerning for HAEC (Table 1.1).[10] Abdominal x-ray may demonstrate gaseous distention of the colon with abrupt cutoff at the level of the pelvic brim—known as "intestinal cut-off sign"—and is both sensitive and specific of HAEC, 74% and 86%, respectively. Other radiological evidence of HAEC include that of enteritis/colitis, toxic megacolon, and pneumatosis intestinalis.[3,5] Free intraabdominal air secondary to perforation may also be present. Children with chronic or recurring HAEC present with persisting diarrhea, intermittent abdominal distention, and failure to thrive. Patients may also present with fever, bloody stools, and vital signs consistent with septic shock. During this period, if there is a concern for abdominal perforation, barium studies and biopsy should be deferred.[1,5]

EMERGENCY DEPARTMENT MANAGEMENT AND TREATMENT

In this case, the parents are becoming increasingly concerned that their child is becoming less responsive and continues to deteriorate. At the top of your differential is HAEC. You assess airway, breathing, and circulation; initiate antipyretics, intravenous fluids, and antibiotics; and order labs and an abdominal x-ray. You inform the parents about your presumed diagnosis, the plan for treatment, and diagnostic evaluation in the emergency department, as well as the possible need for surgical consultation. The

TABLE 1.1. **HAEC Score**

Component	Score
History	
Diarrhea with explosive stool	2
Diarrhea with foul-smelling stool	2
Diarrhea with bloody stool	1
History of enterocolitis	1
Physical Exam	
Explosive discharge of gas and stool on rectal exam	2
Distended abdomen	2
Decreased peripheral perfusion	1
Lethargy	1
Fever	1
Radiologic Exam	
Multiple air fluid levels	1
Dilated loops of bowel	1
Sawtooth appearance with irregular mucosal lining	1
Cutoff sign in rectosigmoid with absence of distal air	1
Pneumatosis	1
Laboratory	
Leukocytosis	1
Shift to left	1
Total	20
	HAEC ≥10

Source: Adopted from Pastor et al.

parents then ask you about what surgery will involve and the long-term implications after treatment.

Emergency department management of patients presenting with signs and symptoms concerning for HD with heightened concern for HAEC should initially begin with assessment and management of airway, breathing, and circulation. Thereafter, intravenous fluid resuscitation, antipyretics, and broad-spectrum antibiotic therapy should be promptly initiated. Frkyman et al. advocate for a 20 mL/kg isotonic fluid bolus followed by 1.5x maintenance fluid replacement during initial resuscitation.[1] For children with persistent, tachycardia and poor perfusion additional fluid boluses should be administered. Ill-appearing children should empirically be started on broad-spectrum antibiotics that provide coverage for enteric gram negative and anaerobes. Ampicillin, gentamycin, and metronidazole triple therapy is an accepted regimen for ill or critically ill appearing patients. *Clostridium difficile* has been associated with HAEC and, should pseudomembranous colitis develop, is associated with a 50% mortality.[3] Patients with known or chronic *C. diff* infections should be supplemented with oral or rectal vancomycin. Unfortunately, studies on comparing the efficacy of a variety of antibiotic regimens are lacking. Ill-appearing patients, or patients with grossly abnormal vital signs, require close hemodynamic monitoring. Patients with a new diagnosis of HD or with concern for HAEC require emergent pediatric surgical consultation as well as prompt pediatric gastrointestinal consultation and follow-up.[1,4]

In consultation with surgery, gastric and enteric decompression should be initiated early. Under direct guidance from pediatric surgery, rectal washout should begin as early as possible with warm normal saline 10–20 mL/kg and may be repeated 2 to 4 times daily until the effluent appears clear. Patients with more severe disease may be at increased risk for abdominal perforation and should have rectal washouts held. In these cases a soft rectal tube should be placed to allow for decompression. In cases of frank vomiting a nasogastric tube should be placed.[1,4,6]

In addition, there is some evidence that sodium cromoglycate, a mast cell stabilizer used commonly in the management of asthma, has been used with some efficacy in some patients in reducing number of bowel movements; however, there are no mutlicenter large-scale studies examining the overall efficacy of these therapies.[1,3]

Definitive management of HD and HAEC is surgical. Though out of scope of practice for emergency medicine providers, a general understanding of the basics of surgical strategies is helpful for discussions with parents and a comprehensive understanding of HD and HAEC. In a broad sense, surgical management aims to resect the abnormal aganglionic segment of bowel and anastomose through to the rectum to normally functioning, ganglionic segments of bowel. The goal is to allow patients to establish regular bowel movements and to maintain continence. Though two-step and multistage open procedures may still be employed by the consulting surgeon, single-stage procedures are gaining favor and are now generally preferred over open techniques.[11] Two common procedures are the Duhamel retrorectal pull-through and the transanal endorectal pull-through (TERPT) procedures. In the TERPT technique, a very low, direct anastomosis is made just above the dentate line, whereas in the Duhamel procedure a side-to-side anastomosis is made between segments of retained aganglionic bowel to a segment of functional ganglionic bowel.[11] A recent article by Arts et al. mention that there is little evidence to support one procedure over the other and that ultimately the surgeon's experience is a key factor in determining the most appropriate procedure as well as postoperative complication rates. Arts et al. suggest that subgroups of patients may benefit from an TERPT as compared to a Duhamel procedure but point out that further evidence and research is warranted.[11] It is important to share with parents and patients that though one-step procedures are preferred, patients with severe HAEC may first require a diverting colostomy, particularly in the setting of abdominal perforation or massively dilated proximal bowel.[1,3,4]

Long-term complications and reports of functionality after surgery are mixed in the literature; some authors cite upward of 90% of patients having normal bowel function after surgery, whereas other studies cite "poor outcomes" in 15% to 30% of cases.[5,6] Though patients with Down syndrome have a higher level of overall mortality associated with HD and HAEC, fecal incontinence and postoperative complication were not more common in patients with Down syndrome, though this may be controversial.[12] Rates of postoperative enterocolitis vary greatly depending on investigator, with some studies citing as low as 0% and others as high as 56%.[13] Recurrent fecal and bowel incontinence apparently increases as age increases, and many adults report persisting problems and issues affecting overall quality of life.[14] In one study by Rintala et al., the authors aimed to explore long-term outcomes in adult and adolescent patients with HD who had corrective surgery in childhood.[14] In their review, bowel function scores indicated that, compared to a normal population, approximately 50% of patients with childhood corrective surgery for HD had lower bowel function scores. In addition, many patients with corrective HD surgery as children will have ongoing and chronic postoperative problems including obstruction secondary to functional aganglionosis, adhesions or strictures, incontinence, and/or recurring episodes of enterocolitis.[14] Repeated episodes of HAEC require further evaluation by surgery. At the discretion of the surgeon, revision procedures including myotomy/ myectomy, botulinum toxin injections, or sphincterotomy may be necessary.[3,5] Despite these shortcomings, according to Moore and Rintala et al., in lieu of patients reporting more social problems relating to incontinence and impaired bowel function compared to control adults, patients with HD appear to be able to be functional members of society and enjoy psychosocial, occupational, and reactional societal norms compared to their peers.[5,14]

It is important to note that studies evaluating the postoperative complications and bowel functions after surgery are often limited by small patient populations, varying severity of aganglionic segments, associated comorbidities, as well as differences in surgical technique.

After adequate volume resuscitation, antibiotic administration, and placing a nasogastric tube, you are able to stabilize your newborn patient. An abdominal radiograph is obtained. You consult general surgery at your hospital; they agree with your concern for HAEC and recommend immediate transfer to the nearest children's hospital for evaluation by pediatric surgery and gastroenterology. You inform the parents of your plan and the need for emergent transfer. They agree to the transfer and are grateful you were able to manage their very ill newborn. You receive word from the pediatric surgeon days later that the surgery was a success and that an excellent outcome is anticpated.

- Any neonate with failure to spontaneously pass meconium in the first 48 hours should be evaluated for Hirschsprung's disease.
- Down syndrome is the most commonly associated congenital abnormality in patients with Hirschsprung's disease.
- Hirschsprung-associated enterocolitis (HAEC) is associated with increased mortality and is associated with abdominal distention, explosive diarrhea, fever, and lethargy. Severe cases will present in shock.
- A HAEC score ≥10 may help aid in diagnosing and evaluating patients with HAEC.
- Abdominal x-ray and barium enema may be helpful in diagnosis; rectal biopsy is the gold standard.
- Patients with a diagnosis of HAEC should receive aggressive fluid resuscitation, broad-spectrum enteric gram negative and anaerobic antibiotic coverage, and close hemodynamic monitoring.
- Cases should be managed with close consultation with pediatric surgery and gastroenterology.
- Definitive management is surgical, with one-step procedures gaining favorability. Severe cases of HAEC may require colostomy.
- Many patients will continue to have bowel impairment later in life despite corrective surgery.

Further Reading

1. Frykman, P., Short, S. (2012) Hirschsprung-associated enterocolitis: prevention and therapy. *Seminars in Pediatric Surgery* 21: 328–335.
2. Swenson, O. (2002). Hirschsprung's disease: a review. *Pediatrics* 109: 914–918.
3. Demehri, F., Halaweish, I., Coran, A., Teitelbaum, D. (2013) Hirschsprung-associated enterocolitis: pathogenesis, treatment and prevention. *Pediatric Surgery International* 29: 873–881.
4. Langer, J., Mattei P. (ed.). (2011) Hirschsprung disease. In *Fundamentals of Pediatric Surgery,* 475–484. New York, NY: Springer.
5. Moore, S. (2016) Hirschsprung disease: current perspectives. *Open Access Surgery* 9: 39–50.

6. Rudolph, C., Benaroch, L. (1995) Hirschsprung disease. *Pediatrics in Review* 16(1): 5–11.

7. Feldman, T., Wershil, B. (2006) In brief: Hirschsprung disease. *Pediatrics in Review* 27(8): e56–e57.

8. Columbo, J., Wassom, M., Rosen, J. (2015) Constipation and encopresis in childhood. *Pediatrics in Review* 36(9): 392–402.

9. Kessmann, J. (2006) Hirschsprung's disease: diagnosis and management. *American Family Physician* 74(8): 1319–1322.

10. Pastor, A., Osman, F., Teitelbaum, D., Caty, M., Langer, J. (2009) Development of a standardized definition for Hirschsprung's associated enterocolitis: a Delphi analysis. *Journal of Pediatric Surgery* 44(1): 251–256.

11. Arts, E., Botden, S., Lacher, M., Sloots, P., Santon, M., Sugarman, I., Wester, T., Blaau, I. (2016) Duhamel versus transanal endorectal pull through (TERPT) for the surgical treatment of Hirschsprung's disease. *Techniques in Coloproctology* 20: 677–682.

12. Wester, T., Lof Gnstrom, A. (2017) Hirschsprung disease—bowel function beyond childhood. *Seminars in Pediatric Surgery* 26: 322–327.

13. Graneli, C., Dahlin, E., Borjesson, A., Arnbjornsson, E., Stenstrom, P. (2017) Diagnosis, symptoms, and outcomes of Hirschsprung's disease from the perspective of gender. *Surgery Research and Practice* 2017: 1–8.

14. Rintala, R., Pakarinen, M. (2012) Long-term outcomes of Hirschsprung's disease. *Seminars in Pediatric Surgery* 21: 331–343.

2 I'm a Hot Baby

Sriram Ramgopal

A 27-day-old former full-term infant, the product of an uncomplicated pregnancy, presents to the emergency department with vomiting, diarrhea, and weight loss for the past 7 days. The parents say that their son has gastroesophageal reflux but that his nonbilious emesis has started to worsen in frequency. They saw their pediatrician at the onset of his symptoms. A stool occult blood test was performed and was positive. The pediatrician recommended a change of formula to an elemental preparation suspecting a diagnosis of milk protein-induced colitis. However, the diarrhea persisted and on the day of presentation, after evaluation with their primary care physician who noted a 1-pound weight loss, he was referred to the emergency department. Vitals are notable for a temperature of 38.6°C and his weight is below the third percentile. The infant has folds of redundant skin, dry oral mucosa, and a capillary refill time of under 2 seconds.

What do you do now?

DISCUSSION

In this previously healthy 27-day-old infant presenting with fever, weight loss, and diarrhea, a careful approach is indicated to evaluate for serious disease. Fever for any reason in an infant under 2 months old requires medical attention, irrespective of the overall appearance of the patient, and often requires a screening evaluation and hospitalization with empiric antimicrobial therapy. Many practice guidelines have distinct recommendations for infants 0 to 28 and 29 to 60 days of age. The management of infants with this common presentation is an area of ongoing research.

A variety of infections can cause a fever in this population. The majority of attention has been in identifying serious bacterial infections (SBIs), a term that includes urinary tract infections (UTIs), bacterial meningitis, and bacteremia and which occasionally includes other entities such as gastroenteritis and consolidative pneumonia. Of all the SBIs, UTIs predominate and are present in 8% to 10% of infants under 60 days of age without localizing symptoms. These are typically caused by *Escherichia coli, Klebsiella, Enterococcus,* and *Enterobacter.* In contrast, rates of bacteremia and bacterial meningitis, which used to be higher in the pre-pneumococcal and Haemophilus influenza vaccination era, are now less common. The incidence of bacteremia and bacterial meningitis is 1 to 2% and 0.5% to 1%, respectively. Common pathogens include Group B Streptococcus, *Escherichia Coli,* and *Staphyloccocus aureus.* Given the less severe and readily identifiable nature of UTIs compared to bacteremia and meningitis, many clinicians have now started to term the latter two as "invasive bacterial infections" (IBIs) to better differentiate these infections from UTIs. Unfortunately, identifying which infants are at greatest risk of IBIs cannot reliably be done by a physical examination alone. Infants with only a history of fever but who are afebrile on vital signs assessment may be at a reduced risk of SBI compared to those who have a documented fever in the emergency department. At best, this likely represents a small risk reduction and should not be used to guide clinical decision-making.

In a febrile infant under 60 days old without a focus of infection on physical examination, a broad workup is typically recommended to identify SBIs. This typically consists of a urinalysis with urine culture, blood culture with complete cell count and differential, and a lumbar puncture for cultures and cell counts. A urinalysis is ideally obtained by a catheterized specimen. Suprapubic aspirations are rarely necessary. Bag specimens, if positive, are unreliable but may be employed as an initial screening test as they can be helpful if negative. A patient having an equivocal or suggestive urinalysis from a bag specimen should have the test repeated from a catheterized sample. A urinalysis with pyuria, positive leukocyte esterase, or nitrite indicates a strong likelihood of UTI. Though a complete blood count with differential is frequently obtained in order to screen for IBI, the value of this test is controversial. One recent large analysis of a multicenter, prospective trial found that the complete white blood cell count has poor discriminatory ability in the identification of infants with IBI. The absolute neutrophil count, while slightly superior in comparison, remains a poor diagnostic test.

As only a small fraction of infants presenting with a fever have an SBI, efforts have been made to risk-stratify infants to identify a cohort at low risk of SBI to allow outpatient management or observation without antibiotics. The first of these efforts was reported in 1988 with the Rochester criteria, which outlined specific lab parameters for the complete blood count, urine, and stool that would identify febrile infants at low risk for SBI. Notably, the Rochester criteria did not require the performance of a lumbar puncture. Since then, updates and refinements to these guidelines, based on ongoing research, further refine low risk criteria for a febrile neonate (Table 2.1). A recently published criterion using multicenter data (the PECARN criteria) does not require use of a lumbar puncture but instead requires only a procalcitonin level, absolute neutrophil count, and urinalysis to risk stratify patients. Infants 29 to 60 days of age who are well appearing and who meet low risk criteria may potentially not require hospitalization or antimicrobial therapy.

In infants, the lumbar puncture can be performed in the lateral recumbent position or sitting upright. Care should be taken to ensure that the infant's hips and shoulders are perpendicular to the examination table. Relying on the gluteal cleft to identify the midline can be misleading. Using a topical anesthetic such as a lidocaine gel can allow for adequate analgesia without obscuring landmarks. A 22-gauge 1.5-inch spinal needle is ideal.

TABLE 2.1. **Low Risk Criteria for a Febrile Neonate**

	Rochester, 1988	Boston, 1992	Philadelphia, 1993	PECARN, 2019
Age	0–60 days	28–89 days	29–56 days	0–60 days
Temperature	≥38.0°C	≥38.0°C	≥38.2°C	≥38.0°C
Historical characteristics	≥37 weeks gestational age Never hospitalized Never treated for hyperbilirubinemia No use of or perinatal exposure to antibiotics No chronic/underlying illness	Caregiver reachable No antibiotics within 2 days No recent immunizations within 2 days No allergies to beta-lactam antibiotics	Presumed to be immunocompetent Reliable and easily reachable caregiver	≥37 weeks gestational age No recent antibiotic use within 4 days No focal infections (except otitis media) Immunocompetent No major congenital abnormality, chronic lung disease, indwelling hardware
Physical examination	Well-appearing	No ear, soft tissue joint, or bone infection Normal vitals, not ill appearing, normal vital signs, well hydrated, taking fluids	Well appearing	Well appearing

Lab characteristics	WBC count 5,000 to 15,000/mm^3 ABC count ≤1,500/mm^3	WBC count <20,000/mm^3	WBC count <15,000/mm^3 Band to neutrophil ratio <0.2	Absolute neutrophil count <4100/mm^3
	Centrifuged UA with ≤10 WBC/hpf	Centrifuged UA with <10 WBC/hpf; negative leukocyte esterase	Centrifuged UA with <10 WBC/hpf and few or no bacteria on Gram stain	UA with ≤5 WBC/hpf; negative leukocyte esterase, urinary nitrite, or pyuria
		CSF with <10 WBC/mm^3	CSF with <8 WBC/mm^3 and negative Gram stain	
		CXR without infiltrate, if indicated	CXR without infiltrate, if indicated	Serum procalcitonin <1.7 ng/ml
	Stool WBC ≤5/hpf (if diarrhea)			

Note: Commonly used risk-stratification guidelines in the United States for the management of young febrile infants. PECARN = Pediatric Emergency Care Applied Research Network; WBC = white blood cell count; ABC = absolute band count, UA = urinalysis; hpf = high-powered field; CSF = cerebrospinal fluid; CXR = chest radiograph; PPV = positive predictive value; NPV = negative predictive value.

The vertebra along the imaginary line connecting the superior iliac crests corresponds to the fourth lumbar vertebrae. After ensuring sterile technique, the needle is inserted between the L3 to L4 or L4 to L5 interspinous process, angled toward the umbilicus and with the bevel pointing towards the ceiling (Figure 2.1). Specimens should be sent for cell counts, culture, protein, and glucose. Interpretation of a traumatic tap (in which cerebral spinal fluid is mixed with frank blood) can be difficult and formula that attempt to correct for the numbers of red blood cells in such a specimen are unreliable.

Beyond UTI, bacteremia, and meningitis, other bacterial infections of significance can lead to fever. Bacterial gastroenteritis can lead to a febrile illness, sometimes associated with bloody stool. In particular, nontyphoidal Salmonella gastroenteritis can be associated with bacteremia. A thorough physical examination can reveal a specific etiology for bacterial infection: a copious eye drainage associated with periorbital swelling may be associated with conjunctivitis, or an erythematous swelling along the medial aspect of the eye may be caused by dacryocystitis. The presence of respiratory symptoms may be secondary to a pneumonia. Cellulitis of the umbilical

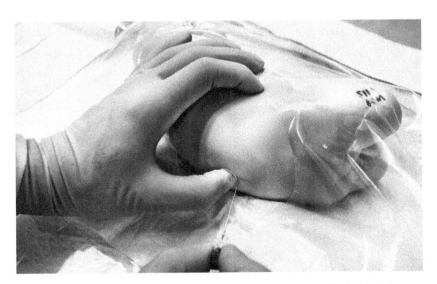

FIGURE 2.1. Performance of a lumbar puncture on a neonate mannequin. The thumb of the nondominant hand is used to palpate landmarks during the procedure.

stump, called omphalitis, should be suspected in the setting of purulent discharge from the umbilicus with surrounding induration, erythema, and tenderness. Even when treated, the mortality rate of omphalitis is high. Soft tissue and joint infections are rare but may be suggested by focal tenderness or unusual positioning.

Viral infections can also cause fever and significant morbidity in these young infants. Agents such as rhinovirus, respiratory syncytial virus, influenza virus, and parainfluenza virus are common. Viral testing for these agents is generally not indicated and, if positive, does not obviate the need for SBI testing. Such infants may require frequent suctioning or supplementary oxygen. Infants are considered to be at high risk for complications of influenza and may therefore warrant antiviral therapy for this infection with oseltamivir. However, data regarding the efficacy of available treatments in this age group are limited.

While the majority of viral infections carry a benign course, special mention should be made of herpes simplex infections. Herpes simplex infections carry significant morbidity and mortality and can be challenging to diagnose. Vertical transmission is less likely in the presence of a cesarean delivery or in cases without a known maternal history of previous herpes infection. The presence of these historical factors alone, however, does not exclude the risk of transmission. Only a minority of patients present with skin, eye and mouth disease, which can be diagnosed by the presence of herpetic vesicles, punched-out erosions, and hemorrhagic crusts, often over an erythematous base. Of those with disseminated or central nervous system disease, approximately one-third do not have any cutaneous findings. Herpesvirus infection should be suspected in an infant with unexplained irritability, sepsis syndrome, or elevated hepatic function tests. Infants with neonatal herpes typically present within 6 weeks of birth. Diagnosis recommendations from the American Academy of Pediatrics require swabs from the mouth, nasopharynx, conjunctivae, and anus for polymerase chain reaction (PCR) assay, specimens from skin vesicles (if present) whole blood and CSF for PCR, and whole blood measurement of alanine transaminase.

The treatment of febrile neonates is guided by the results of physical examination and laboratory findings. Attention to airway, breathing, and circulation are paramount. Ill-appearing infants may benefit from assessment and administration of glucose, if hypoglycemia is present and bolus intravenous fluids, for patients with evidence of hypovolemia. Given the caveats that well-appearing infants may nonetheless have significant disease and the notable limitations in laboratory testing, a cautious approach is recommended, especially in infants less than 1 month of age. Infants who are not low risk following assessment should receive broad-spectrum antimicrobial coverage. A combination of ampicillin with gentamicin or cefotaxime can be used in infants less than 1 month of age, and ceftriaxone (if the postmenstrual age is greater than or equal to 44 weeks) is appropriate for infants between 1 and 2 months of age. Ceftriaxone should not be used in very young infants as it may cause or exacerbate jaundice. Vancomycin can be added if the workup is concerning for meningitis to cover for potential resistant strains of *Streptococcus pneumoniae* meningitis. If herpes virus is considered, empiric acyclovir should also be provided while awaiting the results of confirmatory testing. In general, infants less than 28 days of age should be admitted, whereas infants 29 to 60 days who are well appearing, with reliable caretakers, and who have a complete and normal laboratory evaluation may be candidates for discharge and outpatient therapy.

Given the low rate of IBIs in this population, identifying better ways to risk-stratify infants remains an active area of ongoing research. Given the rarity of meningitis in this population, future recommendations will likely remove the requirement of the lumbar puncture to risk-stratify infants. The measurement of procalcitonin, a proinflammatory biomarker, has been the subject of intense interest as a test to identify those patients at higher risk of IBI. Procalcitonin has demonstrated a superior discriminatory ability compared to C-reactive protein and the complete blood cell count with differential in the identification of invasive bacterial infections. The use of this assay has been incorporated into newer risk-stratification models in Europe and the United States. Further out, a point-of-care test using RNA transcriptional signatures to rapidly determine which patients are at risk of bacterial versus nonbacterial infections may allow for better risk stratification and more judicious use of antimicrobial agents.

For the patient in this vignette, a complete blood count was notable for a white blood cell count of 25,800 cells per microliter, a neutrophil count of 9,550 cells per microliter, and a band count of 4,390 cells per microliter.

Urinalysis was unremarkable. A lumbar puncture was performed with 2 white blood cells per cubic millimeter and no red blood cells. A capillary blood sugar was normal. An abdominal radiograph was normal. The infant was given intravenous fluids to correct dehydration and was empirically treated with ampicillin and gentamicin. He was admitted to the inpatient service, where all cultures were negative. He was diagnosed with viral gastroenteritis and was discharged home after he was able to maintain his hydration orally.

In conclusion, infants under 2 months old with fever present a group of patients with the potential for serious disease. Though the majority are presumed to have viral infections and have a benign course, a careful evaluation for SBI is required. A conservative approach is advised given the high morbidity of these infections and consists of cultures of multiple sites, hospitalization, and empiric antimicrobial therapy. The use of a guideline or clinical pathway in the management of these infants can ensure consistent care.

KEY POINTS

- While the majority of febrile infants less than 60 days old have viral infections with a benign course, a history and physical examination alone cannot reliably exclude SBI in an infant less than 60 days of age.
- For infants less than or equal to 60 days old without evidence of a focal infection, a typical evaluation consists of a urinalysis with urine culture, a complete blood count with differential with blood culture, and a cerebrospinal fluid cell count with culture.
- A conservative approach with hospitalization and systemic antibiotics is advised in infants who do not meet low-risk criteria.

Further Reading

Baker MD, Bell LM, Avner JR. Outpatient management without antibiotics of fever in selected infants. *N Engl J Med*. 1993;329(20):1437–1441. doi:10.1056/NEJM199311113292001

Baskin M, O'Rourke E, Fleisher G. Outpatient treatment of febrile infants 28 to 89 days of age with intramuscular administration of ceftriaxone. *J Pediatr*. 1992;120(1):22–27.

Cruz AT, Mahajan P, Bonsu BK, et al. Accuracy of complete blood cell counts to identify febrile infants 60 days or younger with invasive bacterial infections. *JAMA Pediatr*. 2017;171(11):e172927. doi:10.1001/jamapediatrics.2017.2927

Gomez B, Mintegi S, Bressan S, et al. Validation of the "step-by-step" approach in the management of young febrile infants. *Pediatrics*. 2016;138(2):e20154381. doi:10.1542/peds.2015-4381

Herr SM, Wald ER, Pitetti RD, Choi SS. Enhanced urinalysis improves identification of febrile infants ages 60 days and younger at low risk for serious bacterial illness. *Pediatrics*. 2001;108(4):866–871.

Jaskiewicz J, McCarthy C, Richardson A, et al. Febrile infants at low risk for serious bacterial infection—an appraisal of the Rochester criteria and implications for management. Febrile Infant Collaborative Study Group. *Pediatrics*. 1994;94(3):390–396. doi:10.1542/peds.111.5.964

Kuppermann N, Dayan PS, Levine DA, et al. A clinical prediction rule for stratifying febrile infants 60 days and younger at risk for serious bacterial infections. *JAMA Pediatr*. 2019;173(4):342–351. doi:10.1001/jamapediatrics.2018.5501.

Milcent K, Faesch S, Gras-Le Guen C, et al. Use of procalcitonin assays to predict serious bacterial infection in young febrile infants. *JAMA Pediatr*. 2016;170(1):62. doi:10.1001/jamapediatrics.2015.3210

Watt K, Waddle E, Jhaveri R. Changing epidemiology of serious bacterial infections in febrile infants without localizing signs. *PLoS One*. 2010;5(8):e12448. doi:10.1371/journal.pone.0012448

Woll C, Neuman MI, Pruitt CM, et al. Epidemiology and etiology of invasive bacterial infection in infants ≤60 days old treated in emergency departments. *J Pediatr*. 2018;200:210–217.e1. doi:10.1016/j.jpeds.2018.04.033

3 Shake It Baby

Susana Ho and Melissa A. McGuire

An 11 lb 4 oz baby boy is born to a 29-year-old
obese mother at 35 weeks gestation. The pregnancy
was complicated by maternal gestational diabetes,
while the birth itself was prolonged secondary to
shoulder dystocia. The infant is eventually delivered
via cesarean section. Immediately post-delivery,
the APGAR score is 4. Several breaths are delivered
via bagging and the infant clinically improves to an
APGAR of 8. The next few hours of life are uneventful
for the neonate until 4 hours post-birth when he starts
to become diaphoretic and inconsolable with a weak
cry, and shortly after develops seizure-like activity.
The nonspecific symptoms may represent a large
range of possible pathologies including metabolic,
encephalopathic, infection, congenital, and trauma.

What do you do now?

DISCUSSION

After stabilizing the airway, a capillary glucose level is obtained which comes back at 25 mg/dl, which is confirmed on laboratory blood glucose level. You immediately treat the neonate with glucose and he rapidly returns to baseline mental status. Once you calm the mother down, she rapid fire questions at you. "What happened? Why did this happen? Is this my fault? Could I have prevented this? Will the baby have any long-lasting effects from this?"

Hypoglycemia can present with a myriad of symptoms as exhibited in the presented case. Luckily it is an easily and quickly identified problem. Neonatal hypoglycemia is a distinct entity compared to hypoglycemia in an infant or adult. A neonate has to transition between an exogenous glucose supply via the placenta to endogenous production of glucose based on the neonate's own glucose production capabilities.

The majority of glucose consumption in neonates occurs in the brain. Given their increased head to body ratio as compared to adults, their glucose utilization, 4-6mg/kg/min, is also 2 to 3 times more than an adult. As the primary source of fuel for the rapidly developing brain, much of the concern regarding neonatal hypoglycemia surrounds when hypoglycemia screening should occur, when medical intervention is necessary, and possible downstream neurologic effects of prolonged hypoglycemia.

DEFINITION OF HYPOGLYCEMIA

A strict numerical value of hypoglycemia is a widely debated topic given the lack of correlation between a specific blood glucose value and clinically significant symptoms. Further, there is a lack of data regarding correlations between specific blood glucose levels and neurodevelopmental effects. For example, Neonate A with a blood glucose level of 25 mg/dl may be completely asymptomatic while Neonate B with a level of 40 mg/dl may be seizing from hypoglycemia due to increased rate of glucose utilization. Additionally, there is data showing that treatment of an asymptomatic hypoglycemic newborn is actually detrimental to their neurological development, so there must be careful consideration when it comes to treatment of an asymptomatic neonate. Physiologically, the normal nadir of blood glucose levels in neonates may persist from hours to days after birth without producing symptoms at which point the question becomes: do we treat just the number?

Currently, the American Academy of Pediatrics has defined neonatal hypoglycemia as blood glucose less than 47 mg/dL in the first 48 hours while the Pediatric Endocrine Society has defined neonatal hypoglycemia as blood glucose less than 50 mg/dL in the first 48 hours with a caveat of a level of less than 60 mg/dL in patients where there is concern for congenital hypoglycemia.

EPIDEMIOLOGY/INCIDENCE

Published incidence rates of hypoglycemia vary from 1% to 10% with the incidence of hypoglycemia in at-risk neonates as high as 30%. Risk factors include pre- and post-term infants, infants exposed to conditions causing perinatal stress, infants with intrauterine growth restriction, small and large for gestational age, infants born to diabetic mothers, mothers exposed to beta adrenergic tocolytics, family history of genetic hypoglycemia, congenital syndromes such as Beckwith-Wiedemann syndrome, and erythroblastosis fetalis.

NORMAL PATHOPHYSIOLOGY

Sources of glucose change drastically in utero versus the neonatal period. In utero, a fetus' source of glucose comes from facilitated diffusion via the placenta. This, paired with a fetus's endogenous regulatory system of insulin production, helps to keep the fetus euglycemic. When a fetus is almost full term, there are several mechanisms that help rapidly increase glycogen storage prior to birth. These mechanisms rely on cortisol, insulin, glucose, glucagon, and oxygen levels. Alterations of any of these can cause hypoglycemia in the newborn.

After birth, the neonate must transition to endogenous glycogenolysis and gluconeogenesis as its stored hepatic glycogen is slowly depleted, typically occurring around 8 to 12 hours. Due to this rapid depletion, endogenous glucose production starts around 4 to 6 hours of life and will supply only about 10% of the neonate's glucose. When the newborn receives first feeds, a supply of exogenous glucose helps supplement the neonate's own glucose production. Unfortunately, 10% of full term neonates will become hypoglycemic if feedings are delayed greater than 3 hours after birth.

There are several mechanisms that stimulate neonatal gluconeogenesis and glycogenolysis. One such mechanism is a high glucagon/insulin ratio postpartum, which induces synthesis of the enzymes required for gluconeogenesis. Another is elevated catecholamine levels, which cause the increased release of free fatty acids. This all contributes to the ability to maintain a normal blood glucose level. Any disruptions in these mechanisms or imbalance of substrates can spur hypoglycemia, especially since these mechanisms do not reach maturity until 1 to 2 weeks of age.

In the case of prolonged starvation, the brain can also utilize ketones produced by the liver; however, the preferred source of fuel for the neonatal brain is glucose.

SYMPTOMS

The baby described in our case vignette presented with classic symptoms of hypoglycemia. Symptoms of hypoglycemia are nonspecific but can be separated into either neurogenic versus neuroglycopenic, with neurogenic symptoms typically preceding neuroglycopenic symptoms. Neurogenic, also known as adrenergic or autonomic, symptoms are due to the sympathetic response to hypoglycemia while neuroglycopenic symptoms are due to glucose deprivation of the brain. Neurogenic symptoms present as irritability, sweating, tremors, vomiting, pallor, tachycardia, or tachypnea. Neuroglycopenic symptoms include seizure, lethargy, coma, hypotonia, weak or high-pitched cry, poor feeding, poor suck, vasomotor instability, apnea, bradycardia, hypothermia, and death. See Table 3.1 for common symptoms of hypoglycemia.

CAUSES

Simply put, hypoglycemia is due to the inadequate supply or increased demand of glucose. Causes of hypoglycemia can be broadly categorized into increased utilization versus decreased production. In our case, we presented

TABLE 3.1 Clinical Signs and Symptoms of hypoglycemia

Symptoms associated with autonomic nervous system activation

   Sweating

   Tachycardia

   Nausea, vomiting

   Hypotonia

   Tremor

Symptoms associated with prolonged hypoglycemia

   Lethargy, coma

   Restlessness, Irritability

   Apnea, respiratory distress

   Seizures

a patient with several risk factors for neonatal hypoglycemia including a diabetic mother, hypoxia at birth, prematurity, and large for gestational age.

Hypoxia, prematurity, intrauterine growth restriction, and any causes of intrauterine stress are risk factors for hypoglycemia. Intrauterine stress will increase metabolic demand, thereby increasing glucose utilization. Furthermore, depending on the level of prematurity, the fetus may not have had enough time to build up enough glycogen stores in the last one-third of gestation, as this is when the rapid accumulation of these stores occur. Premature babies also have effects on their hormonal responses to glucose regulation. Newborns that are small for gestational age may not have proper substrate supplies for synthesis of glycogen.

In post-term gestation, multiple gestations, and intrauterine growth restriction, placental insufficiency will cause inadequacy in glycogen diffusion across the placenta, thereby causing hypoglycemia.

With maternal diabetes, there is an excess of glucose diffusion into the fetus's bloodstream, thereby leading to increased insulin secretion in utero. When the baby is delivered, there is still an excess of insulin secreted without the excess supply of glucose. The elevated insulin:glucagon ratio inhibits glycogenolysis, lipolysis, and gluconeogenesis so as the blood glucose is decreasing, there is no glucose production occurring.

Hyperinsulinemia can be caused by a multitude of things including congenital insulinism, maternal use of beta-agonist tocolytics including terbutaline, and erythroblastosis fetalis. In erythroblastosis, an increase in pancreatic beta cells causes an increase in insulin secretion, although the specific cause of the beta cell increase itself is unclear.

Adrenal insufficiency such as congenital adrenal hyperplasia causes neonatal hypoglycemia as cortisol is an important regulatory hormone that stimulates glycogen synthesis. Without the activating effects of cortisol, newborns will develop hypoglycemia. See Table 3.2 for potential etiologies of persistent hypoglycemia, diagnostic testing, and treatment.

SCREENING AND TREATMENT

Recurrent hypoglycemia and hypoglycemic episodes in newborns over 48 hours of life should prompt screening for pathologic causes of hypoglycemia including congenital disorders. Table 3.2 shows the possible etiologies of persistent hypoglycemia.

Physiological hypoglycemia in neonates should have resolved by 48 hours. A newborn's mechanisms for maintaining blood glucose should be further developed and the newborn should have started feeds, thereby helping to maintain his or her blood glucose levels. Blood glucose testing should occur in asymptomatic infants with risk factors such as maternal diabetes, preterm birth, and so on. It should also occur with any infants who are symptomatic. Healthy, at-term, asymptomatic infants should not be tested. All abnormal point-of-care glucose testing should be followed by a lab test given the lack of sensitivities in blood glucose monitors in low and high ranges of glucose.

The management between symptomatic and asymptomatic infants differ. Symptomatic infants should be treated regardless if their blood glucose is 20 mg/dL or 60 mg/dL. Treatment should be started with a bolus of intravenous (IV) dextrose 10% in water (D10W) at 200 mg/kg followed by a continuous infusion. The IV formulation is also first line for infants unable to tolerate oral intake, asymptomatic yet severely hypoglycemic (<25 mg/dL) infants, and in patients with persistent hypoglycemia despite taking oral feeds.

Asymptomatic at-risk infants found to be hypoglycemic should be fed orally. Those at-risk should be orally fed within 1 hour of birth with strict glucose monitoring after feedings.

TABLE 3.2 **Etiologies of Persistent Hypoglycemia, Diagnostic Testing, and Treatment**

Disorder	Clinical Cues	Testing/Diagnosis	Treatment
Inborn Errors - Urea cycle disorders - Organic acidemia - Fatty acid oxidation disorders - Aminoacidurias	Usually presents 12–72 hours of age after initiating oral feeding	Labs Diagnosis: tandem mass spectrometry, typically diagnosed via newborn screen	IV glucose (per normal hypoglycemia protocol) Diet restrictions
Congenital Hyperinsulinemia	Hypoglycemia (≤40 mg/dL) within 1–2 hours of feeding	Labs: Increased plasma insulin and c-peptide (≥0.2 mmol/L) during hypoglycemia, increased glucose requirements, inappropriate glycemic response to glucagon Diagnosis: molecular testing, clinical course consistent with hyperinsulinemia after exclusion of other causes of hyperinsulinemia	IV glucose, diazoxide, stomatostatin analogues such as octreotide. Treatment directed toward decreasing insulin secretion
Beckwith-Wiedeman	Hypoglycemia, hyperinsulinemia, macrosomia, macroglossia, abdominal wall defects, renal abnormalities, hemihypertrophy	No consensus of defined diagnostic criteria. Diagnosis based on presence of characteristic findings. Prenatally, can diagnose via amniocentesis and chorionic villus sampling	
Hypopituitarism/Cortisol/GH deficiency	Pituitary hormone defects present with midline defects (e.g., hypertelorism, cleft lip/palate, microcephallus, cryptochordism) Cortisol deficiency: hypoglycemia, vascular collapse, postural hypotension, tachycardia, fatigue, anorexia, weight loss, eosinophilia GH deficiency: dry skin, baldness, decreased muscle mass, anxiety/depression, temperature sensitivity	Diagnosis based on testing of specific endocrine hormones	Hydrocortisone Levothyroxine GH

Note: IV = intravenous; GH = growth hormone.

LONG-TERM SEQUELAE

Persistent and recurrent neonatal hypoglycemia has detrimental effects on the long-term neurological development of patients. However, it is unclear what the glucose threshold causing these long term neurodevelopmental deficit is. Further, research has shown that treatment of asymptomatic hypoglycemia may cause harm in future neurological development. Given this, more research must be conducted to elucidate when best to treat asymptomatic hypoglycemia.

KEY POINTS

- All neonates undergo a transition in glucose source between the in-utero period and after birth.
- It is important to differentiate normal transient neonatal hypoglycemia from neonatal hypoglycemia from more pathologic causes.
- Do not forget to evaluate for causes of persistent hypoglycemia.
- Treat only symptomatic hypoglycemic and at-risk asymptomatic hypoglycemic neonates with oral or parenteral dextrose.
- Untreated neonatal hypoglycemia may result in negative neurodevelopmental effects in the future.

Further Reading

McGowan J. Neonatal hypoglycemia. *Pediatr Rev.* 1999;20(7):e6–e15. http://pedsinreview.aappublications.org/content/20/7/e6

McKinlay C, Alsweiler J, Ansell J, et al. Neonatal glycemia and neurodevelopmental outcomes at 2 years. *N Engl J Med.* 2015;373(16):1507–1518. doi:10.1056/nejmoa1504909

Rozance P W Jr. Describing hypoglycemia—definition or operational threshold?. *Early Hum Dev.* 2010;86(5):275–280. doi:10.1016/j.earlhumdev.2010.05.002

Rozance P. Management and outcome of neonatal hypoglycemia. Uptodate.com, 2018. https://www.uptodate.com/contents/management-and-outcome-of-neonatal-hypoglycemia

Rozance P. Pathogenesis, screening, and diagnosis of neonatal hypoglycemia. Uptodate.com, 2019. https://www.uptodate.com/contents/pathogenesis-screening-and-diagnosis-of-neonatal-hypoglycemia

Thompson-Branch A, Havranek T. Neonatal hypoglycemia. *Pediatr Rev*. 2017;38(4):147–155. http://pedsinreview.aappublications.org/content/38/4.complete-issue.pdf

Wight N, Marinelli K. ABM Clinical Protocol #1: Guidelines for blood glucose monitoring and treatment of hypoglycemia in term and late-preterm neonates, revised 2014. *Breastfeed Med*. 2014;9(4):173–179. doi:10.1089/bfm.2014.9986

4   Rattled by the Shakes?

Richard Tang and David Foster

A 14-day-old boy, John, is brought in by his parents for intermittent, episodes of right-sided arm and leg twitching and left-sided head turning for the past 2 days with each episode lasting 20 seconds. Initially the episodes occurred only once every few hours but today worsened to 1 to 2 times an hour. He has not been as active as usual. He is formula fed but only fed twice today for a total of 4 oz, much less than his usual 2 to 3 oz every few hours, and only has had one wet diaper today. He has not had any fevers or respiratory symptoms.

He was born at 38.1 weeks. The pregnancy was uncomplicated and the delivery was vaginal. His 4-year old older brother has been coughing for the past few days; there have been no other sick contacts. There is no family history of seizure disorders.

His vitals are: HR 182, RR 50, BP 83/51, SpO2 96%, temp 100.7°F (rectal). Weight is 4 kg.

On exam, John appears tired and unresponsive to the environment. As you begin examining him, he begins to exhibit right-sided arm and leg twitching.

What do you do now?

WHAT ARE NEONATAL SEIZURES?

Seizures are paroxysmal alterations in neurologic function: usually motor, behavior, and/or autonomic function. Neonatal seizures are divided into clonic, tonic, myoclonic, and subtle seizures. Clonic and tonic seizures are further classified into focal and generalized types. However, not all brief episodes of atypical movements and altered mental status are seizures, and care should be taken to avoid misdiagnosis of other conditions with convulsive components. The clinical diagnosis of true seizure activity is often challenging, and studies have shown poor interrater reliability.

Seizures are definitively diagnosed by their electroencephalography (EEG) findings—which are sudden, repetitive, evolving, and stereotyped episodes of abnormal electrographic activity. They can be categorized according to their EEG findings: epileptic (associated with corresponding activity, like clonic seizures), non-epileptic (clinical seizures without corresponding EEG correlate; e.g., subtle and generalized tonic seizures), and EEG seizures (abnormal EEG activity with no clinical correlation).

The diagnosis of seizures is complicated by the fact that less than 20% of electrographic seizure activity is associated with any clinical findings and that clinical signs of seizure activity may resolve upon treatment with antiepileptic drugs, while EEG findings may still persist.

Status epilepticus in pediatric patients, and particularly in neonates, is a common cause of anxiety for emergency medicine providers as a dangerous, complicated, and emergent disease entity. Neonatal status epilepticus is commonly identified as a continuous seizure (or multiple seizures) without a return to baseline neurologic function lasting either for more than 30 minutes or for more than 50% of the total duration of any given period. Many clinicians empirically treat any seizure lasting more than 5 minutes in the emergency department (ED) as a true episode of status epilepticus, similar to pediatric and adult guidelines. Status epilepticus is more difficult to treat and is associated with significantly greater morbidity and mortality relative to non-status neonatal seizures.

HOW PREVALENT ARE NEONATAL SEIZURES? WHAT IS THEIR PROGNOSIS?

The neonatal age group is at highest risk for seizures when compared with other age groups. Approximately 1% of all neonates overall suffer from seizures; preterm neonates are disproportionately affected (up to 20%), while only 0.1% to 0.5% of term neonates are affected. In preterm neonates, the risk of seizure is inversely proportional to both the gestational age (especially < 25 weeks) and birth weight (especially < 1500 g).

There is a high incidence of early death (15% to 20%) associated with neonatal seizures, which largely depends on the severity of the underlying disease process and brain injury. Risk factors for early death include hypoxic-ischemic etiology and high seizure burden. Mortality is even more common among preterm neonates, with mortality rates ranging from 25% to 35%.

Even among survivors, there is an elevated risk of death throughout childhood, and residual motor and cognitive disabilities remain common as well. Furthermore, 20-30% of survivors of neonatal seizures suffer from postneonatal epilepsy, compared with around 1% of the general public.

WHAT IS THE ED MANAGEMENT OF SUSPECTED NEONATAL SEIZURES?

As with the management of any other sick infant, the clinician should adhere to the ABCs of resuscitation, ensuring adequate airway, and cardiovascular support. The clinician should always remember to check a point of care blood glucose early during evaluation, prior to administering any antiepileptic drugs.

Hypoglycemia is difficult to define (generally considered a serum glucose concentration <40 mg/dL in symptomatic term neonates, <45 in asymptomatic neonates, and <30 mg/dL in preterm neonates) and should be emergently managed by providing a bolus of 10% glucose in normal saline, 2 mL/kg IV (200 mg/kg), followed by a continuous infusion of up to 8 mg/kg/min as needed to resolve the hypoglycemia. Additionally, hypocalcemia may be managed with 10% calcium gluconate, 100 mg/kg, followed by a continuous infusion of 500 mg/kg/24 hours, and hypomagnesemia may be treated with magnesium sulfate 25 mg/kg.

The decision of whether to initiate antiseizure drug therapy should be based on multiple factors, including seizure duration, severity, and suspected cause.

The first line treatment of neonatal seizures is phenobarbital (indicated for all children less than 6 months of age), at a dose of 20 mg/kg intravenous (IV; repeated once as needed), followed by a maintenance dose of 4 to 6 mg/kg IV per day, divided into two separate doses. It should be noted that neonates are frequently resistant to initial doses of seizure medications, with an initial treatment failure rate estimated to be up to 50%. It is recommended to rapidly administer a fully adequate loading dose of medication, since patients with fewer seizures are easier to treat in the long term. After resolution of initial seizure activity, it is advised to continue the patient on phenobarbital, 4 to 6 mg/kg/day IV over two divided doses.

If a full dose of phenobarbital has been administered (up to 50 mg/kg/day), but the neonate continues to exhibit seizure activity, second-line agents to be considered are benzodiazepines (midazolam 0.15 mg/kg, lorazepam 0.05–0.1 mg/kg), fosphenytoin (20 mg PE/kg loading dose), levetiracetam (40–60 mg/kg loading dose), or lidocaine (2 mg/kg over 10 min, then 6 mg/kg/hr tapering down over 24 hrs), although there is limited data from randomized controlled trials. Lidocaine and fosphenytoin should be avoided in patients with known cardiovascular pathology, as they can precipitate cardiac dysfunction. Neonatal seizures refractory to phenobarbital often have a limited response to second-line agents.

A midazolam drip (1 mcg/kg/min) may be trialed next if the seizure does not respond to second-line therapy. Otherwise, neonates in status may be empirically trialed on pyridoxine and leucovorin. Bumetanide is a loop diuretic that has limited data showing improved outcomes when given as an adjunct to phenobarbital but has the potential adverse effect of ototoxicity. See Table 4.1.

Acute treatment of neonatal seizures should be continued until all seizures, both clinical and EEG, are controlled. Although antiseizure medications are generally most effective when administered intravenously, there are many other effective options at seizure treatment in

TABLE 4.1. **Treatment Guide for Neonatal Seizures (per IV)**

	Drug	Loading Dose	Infusion rate	Other Doses
First Line	Phenobarbital	20–30 mg/kg	—	50 mg/kg/day max
Second Line	Midazolam	0.15 mg/kg	1 microgram/kg/min	0.4 mg/kg/hr
	Lorazepam	0.05–0.1 mg/kg	—	8 mg/day max
	Fosphenytoin	20 mg PE/kg	100-150 mg PE/min	5–8 mg PE/kg/day maintenance
	Levetiracetam	40–60 mg/kg	—	40–60 mg/kg/day maintenance
	Lidocaine	2 mg/kg	4–6 mg/kg/hr	45 mg/kg/day max
Third Line	(Intubation)	—	—	—
	Pyridoxine	100 mg	—	500 mg/day max
	Leucovorin	2.5 mg	—	—
	Bumetanide	0.05-0.2 mg/kg	—	—

Note: IV = intravenous; PE = phenytoin sodium equivalent units.

patients who do not have IV access. Midazolam is an excellent option, as it has multiple non-IV routes available, including intramuscular, intranasal, and buccal. While fosphenytoin intramuscular (IM) is also another option, its efficacy is greatly diminished relative to its IV administration. Rectal diazepam is a distant third option, as it has a very slow onset of action. See Table 4.2.

While preterm infants have important physiologic and pharmacokinetic differences from term infants and thus may be at higher risk for side effects from antiepileptic therapies, there have been no randomized controlled trials specifically investigating the treatment of preterm neonatal seizures, and there are no guidelines advising for any difference in the acute treatment of their seizures.

TABLE 4.2. **Non-IV Treatment Options for Neonatal Seizures**

Midazolam IM: 0.08 mg/kg
Midazolam IN: 0.3 mg/kg
Midazolam buccal: 0.3 mg/kg
Fosphenytoin IM: 20 mg PE/kg
Diazepam rectal: 0.5 mg/kg

Note. IV = intravenous; IM = intramuscular.

Some neonates may already have a diagnosis of neonatal seizures and/or be prescribed seizure prophylaxis. As antiepleptic drugs (AEDs) may sometimes paradoxically exacerbate seizure activity, if the patient was recently started on an AED, it is safest to avoid administering that medication to the patient.

WHAT COMMON CAUSES OF SEIZURES SHOULD BE CONSIDERED IN THE NEONATE?

There are four broad categories of direct, acute seizure etiologies in neonatal patients—85% of all neonatal seizures are caused by one of these identifiable etiologies, the majority of them are due to acute brain injury.

Hypoxic-ischemic encephalopathies (HIE) are the most common cause of neonatal seizures, and typically present in the first 12 to 24 hours after birth, although they have been found as late as 36 hours. These are especially important to identify early on, as emergent therapeutic hypothermia is vital for treatment. Birth asphyxia is the most common example of this, causing diffuse ischemia and perinatal brain injury. HIE are also associated with high rates of subclinical seizures.

Structural brain lesions are the second most common etiologies of neonatal seizures. Most common in this group is ischemic perinatal stroke, typically involving the middle cerebral artery, which typically manifests as focal clonic seizures. Intracranial hemorrhages may also occur and are commonly caused by trauma, and almost any type can be associated with seizures. Most intracranial hemorrhages can be detected by cranial ultrasound. Preterm infants are at particularly high risk for intraventricular hemorrhage (most common etiology of seizures in preterm neonates). Malformations of cortical development cause less than 5% of all neonatal seizures and include tuberous sclerosis, focal cortical dysplasia, and other rarer disorders.

Transient metabolic disorders should always be excluded as easily reversible causes of seizure activity. Formula overdilution is a classic cause of hyponatremia, and a thorough history of feeding patterns in neonates is always necessary. Hypocalcemia is also a common etiology of neonatal seizures and may be caused by hypoparathyroidism, vitamin D deficiency (often related to the mother's diet or rickets), and hypomagnesemia (which is itself also an independent cause of neonatal seizures). Hypoglycemia is a particularly common etiology of seizures in preterm infants and should always be assessed for early on during the initial clinical presentation. More rarely, inborn errors of metabolism (urea cycles defects, mitochondrial abnormalities, phenylketonuria), maternal narcotic withdrawal, antiquitin deficiency, and PNPO deficiency are additional etiologies but will likely not be diagnosed during the ED management of the neonate.

While older pediatric patients commonly experience simple febrile seizures that carries a benign prognosis, neonatal seizures associated with fever may be caused by *septicemia, with or without central nervous system infections,* and carry a high mortality rate, and neonates should always be investigated with laboratory and imaging studies. Of note, benign febrile seizures are not known to occur to occur in neonates, since they only begin to manifest at 6 months of age.

Especially in neonates with poor prenatal care, the differential diagnosis for infectious etiologies includes TORCH infections (toxoplasmosis, syphilis, rubella, cytomegalovirus, herpes), which are especially common in the perinatal period and can affect up to 2% to 3% of all pregnancies. In such cases with reasonable suspicion for infection, there should be a low threshold to initiate early broad spectrum antibiotic treatment.

Beyond these acute secondary etiologies of seizure, *epilepsy syndromes* cause 15% of all neonatal seizures. Epilepsy is defined as the recurrence of two or more unprovoked seizures. Recurrent seizures in neonates who are otherwise asymptomatic and well appearing are often caused by benign familial neonatal epilepsy, febrile seizures simplex (FSs), acute symptomatic seizures, or benign idiopathic neonatal convulsions (also known as "fifth day fits"). Other epilepsy syndromes with poorer prognosis (and correspondingly ill exams) include early infantile epileptic encephalopathy and early myoclonic encephalopathy.

Benign causes of seizure-like symptoms include breath holding spells and infantile spasms; however, these are rare in neonates and are much more common later in childhood. Benign neonatal sleep myoclonus is another neonatal seizure mimic.

A full history of the seizing neonate should reflect all of these etiologies, focusing on elucidating potential infectious sources, a detailed prenatal and birth history, any possibility of trauma, and any family history of seizure or other neurological disorders. Additionally, the history should closely identify feeding habits, as well as any medications (prescription or over the counter), or supplements the patient may be taking.

WHAT SHOULD THE WORKUP OF NEONATAL SEIZURES INCLUDE?

After the initial resuscitation and stabilization of the seizing neonate, efforts should be made to evaluate for potential seizure etiologies, as listed previously. The evaluation of a neonate requires significantly more testing than older children, secondary to the greater likelihood of an underlying structural, metabolic, or infectious etiology, as discussed in the differential. A point of care glucose should be drawn early upon patient's presentation to rule out hypoglycemia. Laboratory testing should always be obtained in neonates to rule out metabolic abnormalities, particularly hypocalcemia and hyponatremia, which are very common seizure precipitants and easily treated. Less common blood tests that may be considered during the inpatient workup include karyotyping, glycine, ammonia, and long-chain fatty acids. Chest x-rays should be considered in all hypocalcemic patients as part of the evaluation for DiGeorge syndrome.

The physical exam may also be useful to the clinician in providing significant information in the workup of congenital genetic disorders. Patterns of malformations of the hands, eyes, ears, and general head shape may increase the suspicion for fetal alcohol syndrome, for example, and phenylketonuria is commonly accompanied by its distinct musty/mousy odor. Dermatologic findings of nevi, rashes, crusted vesicles, abnormal creases, and hypopigmented patches are also important to note.

The clinician should have a low threshold for evaluating for infections and sepsis causing seizure activity. In addition to a complete blood count, blood culture, and urine culture, a chest x-ray should be included for any respiratory symptoms (cough, congestion, increased work of breathing).

The clinician should have a low threshold to perform a lumbar puncture on any neonate presenting with seizure activity. Certainly, sick or septic appearing infants, or those with persistent neurologic deficits should be considered for lumbar punctures to assess for meningitis or encephalitis; additional considerations for lumbar puncture include a history of lethargy or irritability, decreased oral intake, abnormal appearance, recent antibiotic use, or a positive blood culture. Additionally, any neonate with persistent seizure activity and with unremarkable initial evaluation should be considered for a lumbar puncture, with cerebral spinal fluid (CSF) studies for pleocytosis, xanthochromia, lactic acid, pyruvate, as well as the usual infectious CSF studies.

Neuroimaging is generally not necessary in otherwise healthy neonates who have returned to their baseline after a seizure. However, the clinician should have a low threshold to obtain non contrast cross sectional imaging versus magnetic resonance imaging of the head if the neonate remains lethargic, or generally ill appearing, in order to assess for structural etiologies—particularly ischemic stroke and intracranial hemorrhage. An ultrasound of the fontanelle may also be considered to assess for intraventricular hemorrhages. Neonates who present within the first 48 to 72 hours after birth should be especially considered for hypoxic-ischemic encephalopathy.

All clinical seizures in neonates should undergo further evaluation during an inpatient admission. They should be confirmed by EEG—preferably continuous video-EEG, which is the gold standard of diagnosis. This is especially important as up to 60% of neonates with seizures were found to have one or more subclinical seizures on EEG.

If the patient is already prescribed antiseizure medications, serum drug levels of those medications should be drawn whenever available, even though they may not result until later on during their ED or inpatient stay.

CASE: RESOLUTION

Back to baby John, the 14-day-old who is starting to seize in front of you—what do you do?

Recognizing the critical nature of the situation, a dose of phenobarbital is requested and at the same time a glucose check is ordered. The glucose is 68, a bit low and possibly contributing to the seizure, so you order a dose of D10 at 2 mL/kg. He continues to seize, so a second dose of phenobarbital is administered, which seems to resolve the seizures. He appears lethargic and is minimally responsive to noxious stimulus, although he appears to be protecting his airway at this time, so you choose to monitor him closely and defer intubation at this time. He is placed on cardiorespiratory monitoring, including pulse oximetry and end tidal $CO2$.

Given his functioning diagnosis of status epilepticus, a full septic workup with a complete blood count, comprehensive metabolic panel, chest x-ray, urinalysis, computed tomography of the head, and lumbar puncture is ordered. Additional electrolytes with ionized calcium, magnesium, phosphorus are ordered, and the neurologist is asked to get the patient set up with a stat EEG. The nurse reports that John is starting to twitch again; this time, midazolam is ordered and rapid sequence intubation is initiated. Following the benzodiazepine, he remains intubated and sedated, without any further clinical seizure activity in the ED. John's white blood cell count is 30, and the lumbar puncture shows a high white blood cell count, low glucose, and high protein. The rest of his workup is unremarkable. You send blood cultures, initiate empiric treatment with ampicillin, cefotaxime, and acyclovir, and admit him to the pediatric intensive care unit (PICU).

Later, when you follow up the patient's PICU stay, you find that he grew out group B streptococcus and that he improved over a 2-week admission and was discharged without any seizure medications.

KEY POINTS

- Have a low threshold for a complete metabolic and septic workup in even well-appearing neonates with a first-time seizure or activity suspicious for a seizure.

- Always be prepared for emergent treatment of a seizing neonate: ABCs, glucose, followed by phenobarbital.
- Clinical findings of seizure activity may be subtle in neonates so a high degree of suspicion is required.

Further Reading

Abend, N. S., & Wusthoff, C. J. (2012). Neonatal seizures and status epilepticus. *Journal of Clinical Neurophysiology, 29*(5), 441–448. doi:10.1097/wnp.0b013e31826bd90d

Cornet, M., Sands, T. T., & Cilio, M. R. (2018). Neonatal epilepsies: Clinical management. *Seminars in Fetal and Neonatal Medicine, 23*(3), 204–212. doi:10.1016/j.siny.2018.01.004

Cydulka, R. K. (2018). *Tintinallis emergency medicine manual.* New York: McGraw-Hill Education.

Glass, H. C. (2014). Neonatal seizures. *Clinics in Perinatology, 41*(1), 177–190. doi:10.1016/j.clp.2013.10.004

Glass, H. C., Shellhaas, R. A., Tsuchida, T. N., Chang, T., Wusthoff, C. J., Chu, C. J., . . . Soul, J. S. (2017). Seizures in preterm neonates: A multicenter observational cohort study. *Pediatric Neurology, 72*, 19–24. doi:10.1016/j.pediatrneurol.2017.04.016

Pisani, F., & Pavlidis, E. (2018). What is new: Talk about status epilepticus in the neonatal period. *European Journal of Paediatric Neurology, 22*(5), 757–762. doi:10.1016/j.ejpn.2018.05.009

Pisani, F., & Spagnoli, C. (2018). Acute symptomatic neonatal seizures in preterm neonates: Etiologies and treatments. *Seminars in Fetal and Neonatal Medicine, 23*(3), 191–196. doi:10.1016/j.siny.2017.12.003

Slaughter, L. A., Patel, A. D., & Slaughter, A. L. (2013). Pharmacological treatment of neonatal seizures. *Journal of Child Neurology, 28*(3), 351–364. doi:10.1177/0883073812470734

Soul, J. S. (2018). Acute symptomatic seizures in term neonates: Etiologies and treatments. *Seminars in Fetal and Neonatal Medicine, 23*(3), 183–190. doi:10.1016/j.siny.2018.02.002

5 Those Baby Blues

Tracey Wagner

A 5-month-old female presents to your emergency department via emergency medical services. About 30 minutes prior to presentation she was at home when her parents noticed that she was not breathing normally. They report that her face turned blue. She also seemed to "go limp" in their arms. They called 911 and patted her back. She began breathing and returned to normal. Her parents are not sure how long her symptoms lasted but think no longer than 1 minute. She had eaten 1 hour prior to the event. She has not had any fever, upper respiratory symptoms, or vomiting. She was born at 39 weeks via vaginal delivery without complications. In your emergency department (ED), her vital signs are within normal limits for her age. On exam, she is sleeping comfortably. She easily awakes on your exam and smiles at you. Her heart rate is a regular rate and rhythm without murmur. Her respiratory exam is clear bilaterally. She has no bruises or rashes on full body exam. The remainder of her examination is normal as well.

What do you do now?

BRIEF RESOLVED UNEXPLAINED EVENT

The term "brief resolved unexplained event" (BRUE) was coined by the American Academy of Pediatrics in 2016. It was created to replace a previous diagnosis of "apparent life-threatening event" (ALTE). It defined BRUE as an event occurring in infants younger than 12 months of age who were reported as having a sudden brief episode with at least one of the following symptoms: (a) cyanosis or pallor, (b) absent or irregular breathing, (c) marked change in tone, and/or (d) an altered level of responsiveness. Also there must be no other etiology or diagnosis that better explains the event.

The patient in the vignette provided meets the criteria for BRUE. She is in the proper age range and, notably, has been asymptomatic throughout the entire ED visit. If any symptoms persisted, she could not be classified as a BRUE. In her case, she meets almost all of the associated symptoms of the episode with a change in breathing pattern, a change in color, and a change in tone. Her mental status was not specifically addressed, but to meet criteria for BRUE, only one symptom is required. Peripheral cyanosis such as acrocyanosis or perioral cyanosis or redness are not a valid associated factor. To classify as a BRUE the duration must be less than 1 minute, and this patient's episode was brief. The next step in diagnosing this patient with a BRUE would be to exclude other diagnosis or explanation.

In the majority of cases, excluding other diagnoses may be accomplished with a thorough history, physical exam, and potentially some initial diagnostic testing. During the history ask about any factors that would make an alternative diagnosis, other than BRUE, likely. Other diagnoses to be considered include infection, cardiac abnormality, seizure, choking episode or airway anomaly, reflux, inborn errors of metabolism, or nonaccidental trauma. If the patient history reveals symptoms such as fever, upper respiratory symptoms, respiratory distress, or vomiting, the episode may have been a temporary airway obstruction leading to the event rather than a BRUE. If during the event parents note eye deviation, nystagmus, tonic clonic movements, or spasms, a seizure should be considered in your differential rather than BRUE. Frequently reflux can lead to increased tone and crying. A social history can assist in determining high-risk social situations for nonaccidental trauma.

A thorough systematic comprehensive physical exam should be completed as any abnormal findings can be clues to an alternative diagnosis. On exam, start with vital signs and general appearance, which should be normal with a BRUE. In addition, the patient should exhibit age-appropriate behavior. Infants should have a normal fontanelle without scalp swelling or tenderness to palpation. When examining the eyes, evaluate for normal pupillary responses and for conjunctival hemorrhages. Large amounts of nasal congestion may suggest an upper respiratory infection or temporary airway obstruction. The cardiac rhythm and rate should be within age-appropriate limits, and there should be no cardiac abnormalities. Lung exam should show no increased work of breathing or abnormal breath sounds. A neurologic exam should focus on the patient's response to stimuli, their tone, and symmetry of movement. Evaluate for signs of nonaccidental trauma by closely examining with clothes removed for any skin findings such as bruising or petechiae, indications of tenderness or limited movements of extremities (indicating fracture), tenderness to chest wall (indicating fracture), conjunctival hemorrhages, blood in the nares or oropharynx, or tears to the frenulum.

One of the most concerning differential diagnosis for a BRUE is nonaccidental trauma or child abuse. Bruising is uncommon in infants, especially in those under the age of 5 months, leading to the phrase "those who don't cruise rarely bruise." An additional mnemonic to assist in identifying high-risk bruise patterns includes TEN4FACES. The "T" stands for torso, which includes the chest, abdomen, back, buttocks, and genitals; the "E" stands for ear; and the "N" for neck. The 4 signifies that bruises in these areas should be suspicious in children aged 4 years or younger as well as any bruising in a child 4 months or under. The "FACES" portion further classifies high-risk areas of the frenulum, auricle, cheek, eyelid, and sclera.

After a thorough history and complete examination for exclusion of an alternative diagnosis, the next step is risk stratification to assist in directing further management. Infants with a diagnosis of BRUE must meet several criteria to qualify as lower risk. This should be their first and single BRUE diagnosis. (They cannot have had a previous episode with any of the required features.) They must be greater than 2 months old with a gestational age of 32 weeks or greater and a postconceptional age of 45 weeks or greater. There must also be no concerning exam or history findings. If CPR is performed by a trained medical provider, the patient cannot be classified as lower risk. All criteria must be met for the child to be low risk.

The clinical practice guideline made recommendations for evaluation and management of lower risk infants. ED workup may include pertussis testing, electrocardiogram, and serial observations over 1 to 4 hours. Specifically it recommends against routine testing such as blood work, chest x-ray, EEG, or echocardiograms. Lower risk infants do not have significant increased mortality and can be discharged to home following caregiver education and resources for CPR training. They do not require admission for further monitoring or home pulse oximetry monitoring. Although specific recommendations were not given for higher risk infants, consider further evaluation in the ED and admission to the hospital.

Based on the information provided and presuming the remainder of the history and examination obtained were reassuring and normal, our patient meets criteria for lower risk and could be discharged to home.

KEY POINTS

- The terminology BRUE has replaced ALTE.
- BRUE is defined as an infant less than 1 year of age with a sudden brief, resolved episode with at least one of the following:
  1. cyanosis/pallor
  2. absent, decreased, or irregular breathing
  3. marked change in tone
  4. altered level of responsiveness
- A thorough history and comprehensive exam is necessary to eliminate an alternative diagnosis.
- Lower risk infants with BRUE may be discharged with minimal interventions.

Further Reading

Brand D, Fazzari M. Risk of death in infants who have experienced a brief resolved unexplained event: a meta-analysis. *J Pediatr*. 2018;197:63–67.

McFarlin A. What to do when babies turn blue. *Emerg Med Clin North Am*. 2018;36(2):335–347.

Meyer J, Stensland E, Murzycki J, Gulen C, Evindar A, Cardoso M. Retrospective application of BRUE criteria to patients presenting with ALTE. *Hosp Pediatr*. 2018;8(12):740–745.

Pierce MC, Kaczor K, Aldridge S, O'Flynn J, Lorenz DJ. Bruising characteristics discriminating physical child abuse from accidental trauma. *Pediatrics*. 2010;125(1): 67–74.

Sugar N. Bruises in infants and toddlers. *Arch Pediatr Adolesc Med*. 1999;153(4):399.

Tieder JS, Bonkowsky JL, Etzel RA, et al. Clinical practice guideline: brief resolved unexplained events (formerly apparent life-threatening events) and evaluation of lower-risk infants. *Pediatrics*. 2016;138(2):e20161487.

6 My Broken Heart

Bridget Bonaventura and Beth Bubolz

A 2½-month-old male infant presents with fussiness and poor feeding. Mom says that 2 weeks ago, he began to have trouble feeding. When he starts to feed, he cries, gets fussy and sweaty, and looks pale. Once or twice he seemed to fall asleep after the event. The attacks are getting worse. He has not improved with gastroesophageal reflux treatment or multiple formula changes. The child has a heart rate of 160 bpm, BP 68/40 (right arm), and a O2 saturation of 100%. The infant is well appearing, sleeping, and in no distress. The infant has good color and perfusion. Lung exam reveals rare wheezing bilaterally with no retractions. Heart is a regular rate and mild tachycardia with no murmur. Abdomen is soft with an enlarged liver. You decide it is probably asthma or reflux and give the child an albuterol aerosol. After the breathing treatment you go back to check on the baby and he is trying to feed, but as you are handing the mom the discharge papers, the baby arches away from the bottle in pain. He looks grey, clammy, and sweaty. Then he seems to pass out.

What do you do now?

DISCUSSION

Perhaps rather than WDIDN? (What do I do now?), the question should be WSIHDBIOTDAT? (What should I have done before I ordered that dang albuterol treatment?)

Take a step back and consider the differential diagnosis of a crying baby. Then rethink the history, avoiding all types of bias that might prevent one from considering the dangerous or life-threatening diagnoses. This rethinking should suggest details of the physical exam that will reveal the true diagnosis.

The differential diagnoses may be divided into those that occur *commonly* and those that are *life threatening*. Furthermore, division by organ systems may facilitate recall.

The *commonly* occurring causes of crying in infants may include the following, although it is not an exhaustive list. Most of these conditions can be identified by careful examination or simple testing:

> HEENT: corneal abrasion, foreign body in the eye (eyelash), herpangina, teething or mouth pain. Otitis media.
> ID: URI
> Pulmonary: bronchiolitis
> Gastrointestinal: colic, anal fissure, gastroenteritis, GERD
> GU: testicular torsion, UTI
> Skin/extremities: hair tourniquet

It is critical to consider life-threatening etiologies of crying and use a careful and thorough history and physical exam to exclude them in a logical manner; a systematic approach by organ system is helpful. The clues to detecting these are present, but the examiner must be looking for findings to suggest a serious condition in order not to be blinded.

> Gastrointestinal: Intussusception, volvulus, incarcerated hernia.
> Neurologic: Head trauma, skull fracture, subdural hematoma, or child abuse. As a side note, crying is a risk factor for child abuse. Also in the differential are seizures, meningitis.
> Skeletal: Occult fracture/child abuse.
> Metabolic/Toxic: Hypoglycemia, electrolyte abnormalities, other inborn errors of metabolism, toxic exposure, neonatal abstinence.

Pulmonary: Bronchiolitis, pneumonia, asthma.

Cardiac: Any of the cardiac diagnoses which cause excessive crying are potentially life threatening. These include congestive heart failure (CHF) or dilated cardiomyopathy (DCM) due to any cause. Consider arrhythmias such as supraventricular or ventricular tachycardia, complete heart block, or symptomatic bradycardia. Long QT syndrome will not cause fussiness but could be responsible for "passing out" or "falling asleep" after an attack. Coarctation of the aorta may present with subtle signs of poor feeding but usually occurs a little earlier when the ductus arteriosus closes (first 2 weeks of life). Four extremity blood pressures (arm and leg blood pressures), checking for pulse discrepancies, between upper and lower extremities will alert the astute examiner to this diagnosis. Anomalous left coronary artery arising from the pulmonary artery (ALCAPA) typically presents around 10 weeks of life (range 2–3 months) concurrent with the fall in pulmonary vascular resistance (PVR). Symptoms are due to cardiac ischemia that occur with the stress of feeding.

A thorough evaluation of a crying infant should include both common and life-threatening etiologies. This infant most likely has a cardiac etiology for the crying.

Key features that implicate cardiac disease are sweating and fussiness precipitated by feeds and the age of the patient. The only physical findings to suggest the diagnosis include tachypnea, tachycardia, wheezing, hepato-megaly, and possibly PMI displacement of the point of maximal impulse of the left ventricle. Late findings would include a murmur or gallop.

Feeding is the most vigorous activity that an infant does. It is the equivalent to exercise in an older child or adult. The association of sweating and pallor with feeding in a baby points to a cardiac cause much like symptoms with exertion suggest inadequate cardiac output in an adult. Difficulty feeding opens the whole array of potential cardiac diagnoses, including coarctation of the aorta, cardiomyopathy, ventricular septal defect, arrhythmia, and so on.

Abnormal vital signs document tachypnea and tachycardia. Blood pressure in the right arm is normal, likely ruling out coarctation of the aorta which usually results in hypertension of the upper extremities and at least 30 mm Hg lower BP in the lower extremities. Pressure overload on the left ventricle due to coarctation of the aorta may cause CHF or DCM, as the young heart does not tolerate the pressure overload well. Therefore, checking the femoral pulse is an important part of the complete exam.

Wheezing may be due to many causes and a cardiac cause for wheezing should always be considered. Remember all wheezes are not asthma! Also, checking for hepatomegaly is key to discerning CHF. This must be done by careful palpation starting in the pelvis and slowly, gently working toward the chest. If palpation is not possible, consider placing a stethoscope over the liver and scratching gently on the skin in a mid-clavicular line to hear where the scratching sound changes from sounding solid (over the liver) to sounding hollow (over the intestine) in order to estimate the liver span.

Following a diagnostic evaluation this infant was diagnosed with an anomalous left coronary artery arising from the pulmonary artery.

What is happening physiologically? The timing of this child's symptoms coincide with a decrease in pulmonary vascular resistance (PVR). At birth PVR is high, but it falls over the first 2 months due to regression of smooth muscle hypertrophy (which is necessary in utero). This results in lower pressure in the pulmonary artery and translates to poor perfusion of the left coronary artery (LCA) if it arises from the pulmonary artery. Thus when stressed (e.g., with feeding), the LCA, which is now inadequately perfused with cyanotic blood, cannot meet the metabolic demands of the left ventricular myocardium. The result is ischemia, pain, and the observed clinical signs of sweating and pallor.

An anomalous left coronary artery arising from the pulmonary artery is eponymously known as Bland-White-Garland syndrome for the doctors at Massachusetts General Hospital who described the condition in 1933. (This is the same Paul Dudley White who described Wolff Parkinson White syndrome.)

The best next steps for this infant would be to hold the feeds and place the child on cardiac and pulse oximetry monitors. If the baby does not recover consciousness after the albuterol nebulizer treatment, initiate resuscitation; most likely the arrest is secondary to cardiac ischemia or ventricular tachycardia (VT) due to the former. If the child recovers from the spell, consider supplemental oxygen. Check the glucose and obtain an EKG and chest x-ray. Keep the baby as calm as possible. Avoid intravenous placement or venipuncture. Call the local pediatric cardiologist as soon as EKG and chest x-ray results are available.

Chest x-ray typically shows an enlarged cardiac silhouette due to ischemic dilated cardiomyopathy with ALCAPA, but there are reports of normal heart size. This child's x-ray shows an enlarged cardiac silhouette. Invariably, the EKG is reported as abnormal. This child's ECG is shown Figure 6.1. The classic findings include abnormal Q waves in I, aVL, V5, and V6. Some patients do not exhibit abnormal Q waves, or the finding is transient. In these cases, look for an abnormal R wave progression, low voltage QRS complexes, T wave abnormalities, or ST segment elevation or depression. This child should be admitted to the cardiac intensive care unit on telemetry. He was found to have ALCAPA and was admitted and underwent surgical correction of the abnormal coronary artery.

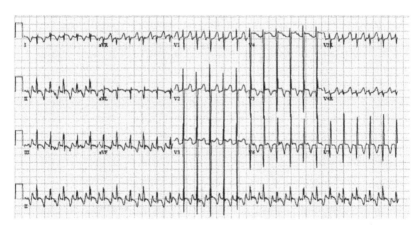

FIGURE 6.1   EKG demonstrates Sinus tachycardia, widespread T wave inversions, ST elevation in V3-6 with Q waves in V5 and V6 and poor R wave progression.

- Cardiac disease in infants typically presents when the arterial duct closes (first 2 weeks of life) or when the pulmonary vascular resistance falls (around 2 months of life).
- Difficulty feeding, abnormal breathing, sweating with feeds, or fussiness may all be presenting symptoms of babies with heart problems.
- Do not miss an enlarged liver by palpating too high in an infant. Start palpating in the pelvis and work toward the chest. Other essential components of the cardiac exam in an infant are careful auscultation over chest and back and palpation of femoral and brachial pulses.
- Feeding is like running a marathon for a baby. Feeding = exercise!
- Initial workup for cardiac disease should always include an electrocardiogram and chest x-ray.

Further Reading

Agrawal H, Mery CM, Sexson Tejtel SK, et al. Familial clustering of cardiac conditions in patients with anomalous aortic origin of a coronary artery and myocardial bridges. *Cardiol Young*. 2018;28(9):1099–1105.

Allen DR, Schieken RM, Donofrio MT. Hoarseness as the initial clinical presentation of anomalous left coronary artery from the pulmonary artery. *Pediatr Cardiol*. 2005;26(5):668–671.

Bland EF, White PD, Garland J. Congenital anomalies of the coronary arteries: Report of an unusual case associated with cardiac hypertrophy. *Am Heart J*. 1933;8(6):787–801.

Dolbec K, Mick NW. Congenital heart disease. *Emerg Med Clin North Am*. 2011;29(4):811–827, vii.

Guzeltas A, Ozturk E, Tanidir IC, Kasar T, Haydin S. Evaluation of anomalous coronary arteries from the pulmonary artery. *Braz J Cardiovasc Surg*. 2017;32(1):29–37.

Hoffman JI. Electrocardiogram of anomalous left coronary artery from the pulmonary artery in infants. *Pediatr Cardiol*. 2013;34(3):489–491.

Judge P, Meckler G. Congenital heart disease in pediatric patients: recognizing the undiagnosed and managing complications in the emergency department. *Pediatr Emerg Med Pract*. 2016;13(5):1–28.

Levitas A, Krymko H, Ioffe V, Zalzstein E, Broides A. Anomalous left coronary artery from the pulmonary artery in infants and toddlers misdiagnosed as myocarditis. *Pediatr Emerg Care*. 2016;32(4):232–234.

Mazurak M, Kusa J. The radiologist's tragedy, or Bland-White-Garland syndrome (BWGS). On the 80(th) anniversary of the first clinical description of ALCAPA (anomalous left coronary artery from the pulmonary artery). *Kardiochir Torakochirurgia Pol*. 2014;11(2):225–229.

Özdemir R, Karadeniz C, Demirpençe S, Doksöz Ö, Yozgat Y, Meşe T. A rare cause of respiratory distress in the emergency department: anomalous origin of the left coronary artery from the pulmonary artery. *Pediatr Emerg Care*. 2015;31(5):357–359.

Patel SG, Frommelt MA, Frommelt PC, Kutty S, Cramer JW. Echocardiographic diagnosis, surgical treatment, and outcomes of anomalous left coronary artery from the pulmonary artery. *J Am Soc Echocardiogr*. 2017;30(9):896–903.

Shaahinfar A, Ghazi-askar ZM, Siroker H, Nagdev A. Anomalous left coronary artery from the pulmonary artery presenting as dilated cardiomyopathy with regional wall motion abnormality on point-of-care ultrasound. *Pediatr Emerg Care*. 2019; 1–3.

Wampole AJ, Hagen SA, Peterson AL. Symptomatic presentation of an anamalous left coronary artery from the pulmonary artery in an 8-day-old. *Pediatr Emerg Care*. 2016;32(5):326–328.

Willner EL, Patel S. Crying. In: Bachur R. *Fleisher & Ludwig's Textbook of Pediatric Emergency Medicine*. 7th ed. Philadelphia: Wolters Kluwer; 2015:121–122.

7 Hot and Bothered

Christopher Perry and
Nechama Sonenthal

A mother brings her infant son to the emergency
department after she noticed the child "was
acting fussy" and "felt warm" this evening. The
child was born 6 weeks ago, full term, after an
uncomplicated vaginal delivery, and has received all
of his scheduled immunizations. The mother noted
his rectal temperature was 38.4°C. She gave him
acetaminophen about 30 minutes ago, and the child is
now afebrile and back to his baseline playful activity
level. According to his mother, he has been feeding
well and gaining weight appropriately. He has had no
other medical problems prior to this and has never
been treated with antibiotics. Apart from the fever, his
review of systems is entirely unremarkable. On your
exam, his vital signs are within normal limits, and the
child is well-appearing, playful, with normal tympanic
membranes, a normal appearing oropharynx, clear
lungs, a soft non-tender abdomen, and no abnormal
skin, bone, or joint findings.

What do you do now?

FEVER IN A WELL-APPEARING INFANT

This child's presentation represents a very common, yet extremely challenging, scenario faced regularly by emergency physicians. Fever is the most frequent chief complaint for children under the age of 15 years presenting to emergency departments in the United States (1). Differentiating between those with a benign viral illness and those with a serious bacterial infection (SBI) or a serious viral infection, such as herpes simplex virus, is essential. This is particularly true for children under 3 months of age given their relatively immature immune systems. Up to 9% (2) of such patients, even if well-appearing, may have an SBI, which could lead to grave long-term sequelae if left untreated. Complicating the issue further is the changing prevalence of invasive organisms with modern vaccine schedules (3–6, 12).

Despite the unremarkable history and the benign physical exam, there is still cause for concern with this child. In infants under 3 months of age, clinical exam and history alone are not sufficiently reliable to exclude an SBI (2, 7, 8). Additionally, the child received an antipyretic prior to coming to the hospital, potentially masking a fever on presentation to the emergency department. The improvement in his fever in response to acetaminophen does not rule out the possibility of an SBI (10, 11). Further work-up is therefore warranted, and the child may possibly need empiric antibiotics and admission.

The initial history and exam is the first step in identifying whether significant risk factors exist for an SBI. The age of this child is important, as the risk for SBI in an infant is inversely related to their age, with the highest rates in the first month of life (8, 9). An immunization history must also be elicited, as immunization with pneumococcal and Haemophilus influenzas type B (HiB) vaccines have been shown to significantly lower the risk of SBI in children (3–6, 12). The absolute temperature needs to be taken into account, as hyperpyrexia (rectal temp greater than 40°C) has been demonstrated to increase the likelihood of SBI (13). Other features in the history which, if present, could point to a higher risk of SBI include prematurity, comorbidities, chronic illness, and recent (within prior week) use of antibiotics.

A full sepsis evaluation should be undertaken if a child meets any of these high risk features or for any child who is ill-appearing or who is under 4 weeks of age. A full sepsis work-up is also indicated if the infant has findings suggestive of HSV infection, such as mucocutaneous vesicles, seizures, or focal neurological findings. The child in our current scenario does not meet any of these high-risk features, but SBI remains a concern due to his age. Further evaluation is therefore required.

The specific work-up for this child will vary to some degree based on clinician judgment and the local practices of the institution where one practices. However, a number of evidence-based guidelines and clinical prediction models have been developed to help guide the clinician in this decision process.

These models (the Boston, Philadelphia, Rochester criteria and PECARN) are summarized in Table 2.1 in the neonatal fever chapter.

Such clinical prediction rules may also need to be reassessed and modified given the changes in prevalence of SBIs in the post-vaccination era. Vaccines, herd immunity, and prenatal Group B strep prophylaxis have decreased the risk of SBIs over the past several decades (3–6, 12), and clinical tools, to be effective, should reflect such changes. However, in the absence of large-scale studies examining such differences, practices for infants under the age of 3 months should not yet change based on post-vaccine prevalence alone.

Beyond these clinical prediction rules, novel diagnostic tests are also finding an increasing role in the workup of pediatric fever. Such tests, including C-reactive protein (CRP) and procalcitonin (PCT), when used either in conjunction with established criteria or as part of a "step-by-step" approach, may have potential to improve accuracy in diagnosis of SBIs.

CRP is an acute phase reactant that rises within 4 to 6 hours after onset of inflammation or tissue injury (23) and declines rapidly on resolution of the inflammatory process. Due to the rapid kinetics involved in its metabolism, it has gained widespread use in medicine as a measure of acute disease activity among a broad spectrum of patient populations. Among neonates, despite the immaturity of their immune system, CRP has been shown to be produced hepatically in response to acute inflammation (24) and is not seen to cross the placenta in appreciable quantities (23, 24), making it potentially attractive as a marker for neonatal sepsis.

Unfortunately, CRP alone has not been shown to have a high enough sensitivity or negative predictive value to be relied upon in isolation to determine the presence of a serious or invasive bacterial infection in neonates (25, 26). However, CRP's association with inflammation, particularly secondary to bacterial infection, may be useful in guiding treatment for neonatal fevers, especially when trending CRP values to assess progression of infection in response to treatment (23).

PCT, the pro-hormone of calcitonin, can increase by hundreds- to thousands-fold in response to systemic bacterial infection (43) and, like CRP, has been studied as a potentially accurate marker for identification of SBIs among febrile infants presenting to the emergency department. Multiple studies (25, 38, 39, 40, 42) have demonstrated superiority to white blood count (WBC) and to CRP for identifying SBI among febrile infants, with at least one study yielding a negative predictive value for PCT of 96.1% (37). A significant heterogeneity does exist among the studies (43), limiting the applicability to the subset of patients between 0 to 90 days who are otherwise well-appearing. And even the highest negative predictive values found would still lead to an unacceptable number of infant SBIs going undiagnosed. PCT thus remains unsatisfactory as an isolated test to rule out SBI in febrile infants.

However, despite being insufficient to rule out SBI when taken independently, such lab tests have shown promise when used in combination with each other or as part of a stepwise approach.

The "step-by-step" approach was created as an algorithm for identifying febrile infants who could be safely managed as outpatients without the need for empiric antibiotics or LP (30, 31). The approach begins with the general appearance of the infant and then sequentially assesses the age, the results of the urinalysis, and the results of biomarkers including PCT, CRP, and absolute neutrophil count (Table 7.1). This approach has been shown to have a higher sensitivity (92.0%) and negative predictive value (99.3%) than the Rochester criteria, while still avoiding the need for routine LP. Of note, the age cut-off for the step-by-step approach was 21 days based on previous studies that indicated this was more appropriate than the classical guideline of 28 days (32). However, 4 of the 7 patients in the Gomez et al. study (out of 2,185 patients evaluated overall) identified as low risk but

TABLE 7.1. **High-Risk Criteria Using Step-by-Step Approach**

Abnormal Pediatric Assessment at Triage or Ill Appearance

Age < or = 21 days old

Leukocyturia

PCT > or = 0.5 ng/ml

CRP > 20 mg/L or ANC >10,000/mm^3

Note. If none of the above criteria are met, patient can be classified as "low risk."
PCT = procalcitonin; CRP = C-reactive protein; ANC = absolute neutrophil count.
Source. Adopted from Gomez et al.[30]

eventually diagnosed with an IBI, were between the ages of 22 and 28 days (30), suggesting that the 28-day cut-off may still be more appropriate.

Although the step-by-step approach has the benefit of identifying low-risk patients without the need for chest x-ray (CXR), LP, or stool studies, it does not give guidance on when to check these studies if an infant is classified as high risk. The question of when to perform an LP, in particular, remains an area of significant debate and controversy. A theoretical concern in giving patients antibiotics without checking an LP is that it could lead to incomplete treatment of meningitis. Until further research provides more definitive answers, an LP should be performed on all infants deemed high risk based on clinical judgment or on criteria such as the step-by-step approach. However, it is reasonable to defer a CXR if the patient does not have respiratory symptoms or findings and to not perform stool studies if the infant does not have diarrhea.

Similarly, the step-by-step approach, as with other criteria, does not offer guidance on whether high-risk patients require admission. However, as with the question of performing an LP, in the absence of large-scale studies demonstrating otherwise, all high-risk infants should likely be admitted for close observation and treatment with empiric antibiotics.

Recommendations for which antibiotics to use for empiric treatment of high-risk infants is given in Table 7.2.

Applying the step-by-step approach to the child in our scenario, the general appearance was first assessed and the child was determined to be well-appearing. Our child did not meet the "high-risk" age of less than 21 days,

TABLE 7.2. **Recommended Empiric Antibiotic Therapy for Febrile Infants Under 36 Months**

Age/Findings	Therapy
Younger Than One Month	Ampicillin* (100 to 200 mg per kg per day IV or IM divided every six hours) plus gentamicin† (2.5 mg per kg IV or IM every eight hours, with adjustments based on serum levels) Alternative: ampicillin* (100 to 200 mg per kg per day IV or IM divided every six hours) plus cefotaxime (Claforan; 50 mg per kg IV every eight hours)
Older Than One Month, Urinary Findings	Cefotaxime* (50 mg per kg IV every 8 hours) Alternative: cefixime‡ (Suprax; 8 mg per kg twice on first day, then 8 mg per kg daily)
One to Three Months, Meningitis Not Suspected	Ceftriaxone (Rocephin; 50 mg per kg per day IV or IM divided every 12 to 24 hours)
One to Three Months, Meningitis is a Concern	Ceftriaxone (100 mg per kg per day IV or IM divided every 12 to 24 hours) Add vancomycin if S pneumonia suspected to cover for resistant strains
One to Three Months, Listeria or Enterococcus is a Concern	Add ampicillin* (100 to 200 mg per kg per day IV or IM divided every 6 hours) to other antibiotics

Note. IM = intramuscularly; IV = intravenously.
*Dosage for children older than 7 days who weigh more than 2,000 g.
†Dosage for children older than 7 days.
‡Cefixime therapy in children younger than 6 months is an off-label use.
Source. Adapted from Hamilton et al.[45]

or even 28 days if that is the criterion used. Urinalysis was then checked, which was negative, including no leukocyturia. Proceeding along the algorithm, blood work was drawn and included blood cultures, complete blood count (CBC) with differential, PCT, and CRP. In our patient, the PCT level was 0.8 ng/ml, which placed him in the "high risk" category. Given this, an LP was performed, which showed no pleocytosis. As he had no respiratory symptoms or findings, a CXR was not checked. He was then given ceftriaxone 50 mg/kg and admitted.

After 48 hours in the hospital, the child's blood, urine, and CSF cultures were negative and he remained afebrile and well appearing. He was then discharged home in stable condition.

CHILDREN 3 TO 36 MONTHS

Had the child in our scenario been between 3 months and 3 years of age, a different management plan would be indicated. Children in this age group have more mature immune systems than infants and have also generally received a higher proportion of their childhood vaccines. They are also somewhat less challenging with regard to history and physical exam than infants, although they still present many difficulties.

Clinical practice varies widely with this age group, with up to 58% of patients not receiving any diagnostic testing whatsoever (33). Much of this variability has been due to the growing data and evolving evidence since the advent of widespread vaccination against Haemophilus influenzas type B (HiB) and Streptococcus pneumoniae (PCV7 or PCV13). A cost effective analysis in 2001 (46) concluded that if the rate of occult bacteremia in this age group were to decline to less than 0.5%, then a "clinical judgement" approach (i.e., eliminating the use of empiric testing or treatment) would be appropriate.

Given that multiple studies (48, 49, 50, 51) have in fact demonstrated such low rates of bacteremia in well-appearing fully vaccinated febrile children in this age group, many experts are now advocating a noninvasive strategy (i.e., no blood draw and no empiric antibiotics) in their management (47, 48).

Urine testing should be considered for febrile children in this age group deemed to be at high risk for urinary tract infection. Baraff et al. in 2008 recommended that a urinalysis and urine culture be checked for girls younger than 2 years, uncircumcised boys younger than 2 years, and circumcised boys younger than 6 months (35). The American College of Emergency Physicians 2016 guidelines (34) recommend consideration of urinalysis and urine culture for well-appearing children aged 2 months to 2 years with a fever, especially among those with high risk features, which includes females younger than 12 months, uncircumcised males, nonblack race, fever duration greater than 24 hours, higher fever (greater than or equal to≥39°C), negative test result for respiratory pathogens, and no obvious source of infection.

Unvaccinated children, as well as those (such as those under the age of 6 months) who have not completed their vaccine schedules for HiB and PCV7 or PCV13, should not be managed with this assumption of a low incidence of bacteremia. A reasonable approach would be to begin with CBC and blood cultures, as well as urinalysis and urine culture for those considered high risk as detailed earlier. Those with WBC greater than 15,000 should be empirically treated with antibiotics and have blood cultures sent. The decision to admit versus discharge home with 24-hour follow-up should be at the discretion of the clinician and should factor into account the appearance of the child as well as the reliability of the child's caregivers.

As is the case with infants, any toxic-appearing febrile child in this age group without an obvious source of infection should undergo a full sepsis evaluation and be treated accordingly.

CHILDREN OLDER THAN 3 YEARS

Children above the age of 3 years who have received all of their vaccines represent less of a diagnostic challenge than younger children, as a more thorough history and physical exam is possible, and also due to the fact that they have significantly more mature immune systems. However, very limited data exists on the management of febrile children at this age who have not received their vaccinations. Assessment and management of febrile patients in this age group should be guided by the specific situation and by the clinical discretion of the practitioner, with a higher degree of concern given to those children who are either ill appearing or who have not received their vaccines.

CONCLUSION

Pediatric fever represents a very common yet incredibly challenging clinical scenario faced daily by emergency physicians. With the advent of widespread vaccinations against common pathogens, and with the development of more advanced diagnostic testing strategies, the assessment and management of such patients continues to evolve. However, clinical judgment remains the clinician's most important tool and must always take into account many factors including age and other historical and physical exam features. When in doubt, always exercise the highest degree of caution that the patient may have an SBI or other serious pathology.

KEY POINTS

. Excluding an SBI is essential for a child under 3 months of age presenting with fever.
. For infants between 28 days and 90 days of age, the "step-by-step" approach has been demonstrated to have superior sensitivity and negative predictive value compared to classic guidelines with regard to identifying infants at high risk for SBI.
. Febrile infants deemed to be high risk for SBI should receive empiric antibiotics and be admitted for close observation.
. Recommendations continue to evolve with changing prevalence of SBI in the post-vaccination era.

Further Reading
1. National Center for Health Statistics. 2011 National Hospital Ambulatory Medical Care Survey, ED summary table 10—Ten leading principal reasons for emergency department visits, by patient age and sex: United States, 2011. https://www.cdc.gov/nchs/data/ahcd/nhamcs_emergency/2011_ed_web_tables.pdf
2. Slater M, Krug SE. Evaluation of the infant with fever without source: an evidence based approach. *Emerg Med Clin North Am*. 1999;17:97–126, viii–ix.
3. Watt K, Waddle E, Jhaveri R. Changing epidemiology of serious bacterial infections in febrile infants without localizing signs. *PLoS One*. 2010;5:e12448.

4. Rudinsky SL, Carstairs KL, Reardon JM, et al. Serious bacterial infections in febrile infants in the post-pneumococcal conjugate vaccine era. *Acad Emerg Med*. 2009;16:585–590.

5. Lee GM, Harper MB. Risk of bacteremia for febrile young children in the post-Haemophilus influenzae type B era. *Arch Pediatr Adolesc Med*. 1998;152:624–628.

6. Whitney CG, Farley MM, Hadler J, et al. Decline in invasive pneumococcal disease after the introduction of protein-polysaccharide conjugate vaccine. *N Engl J Med*. 2003;348:1737–1746.

7. Baker MD, Avner JR, Bell LM. Failure of infant observation scales in detecting serious illness in febrile, 4- to 8-week-old infants. *Pediatrics*. 1990;85:1040–1043.

8. Pantell RH, Newman TB, Bernzweig J, et al. Management and outcomes of care of fever in early infancy. *JAMA*. 2004;291:1203–1210.

9. Bachur RG, Harper MB. Predictive model for serious bacterial infections among infants younger than 3 months of age. *Pediatrics*. 2001 Aug;108(2):311–316.

10. Bonadio WA, Bellomo T, Brady W, et al. Correlating changes in body temperature with infectious outcome in febrile children who receive acetaminophen. *Clin Pediatr*. 1993;32:343–346.

11. Baker MD, Fosarelli PD, Carpenter RO Childhood fever: correlation of diagnosis with temperature response to acetaminophen. *Pediatrics*. 1987;80:315–318.

12. Carstairs KL, Tanen DA, Johnson AS, Kailes SB, Riffenburgh RH. Pneumococcal bacteremia in febrile infants presenting to the emergency department before and after the introduction of the heptavalent pneumococcal vaccine. *Ann Emerg Med*. 2007 Jun;49(6):772–777.

13. Stanley R, Pagon Z, Bachur R. Hyperpyrexia among infants younger than 3 months. *Pediatr Emerg Care*. 2005 May;21(5):291–294.

14. Hui C, Neto G, Tsertsvadze A, et al. Diagnosis and management of febrile infants (0–3 months). *Evid Rep Technol Assess (Full Rep)*. 2012;205:1–297.

15. Baker MD, Bell LM, Avner JR. Outpatient management without antibiotics of fever in selected infants. *N Engl J Med*. 1993;329:1437–1441.

16. Baskin MN, O'Rpourke EJ, Fleisher GR. Outpatient treatment of febrile infants 28 to 89 days of age with intramuscular administration of ceftriaxone. *J Pediatr*. 1992 Jan;120(1):22–27.

17. Kaplan RL, Harper MB, Baskin MN, Macone AB, Mandi KD. Time to detection of positive cultures in 28- to 90-day-old febrile infants. *Pediatrics*. 2000 Dec;106(6):E74.

18. Dagan R, Powell KR, Hall CB, Menegus MA. Identification of infants unlikely to have serious bacterial infection although hospitalized for suspected sepsis. *J Pediatr*. 1985 Dec;107(6):855–860.

19. Dagan R, Sofer S, Phillip M, Shachak E. Ambulatory care of febrile infants younger than 2 months of age classified as being at low risk for having serious bacterial infections. *J Pediatr*. 1988 Mar;112(3):355–360.

20. Jaskiewicz JA, McCarthy CA, Richardson AC, White KC, Fisher DJ, Dagan R, Powell KR. Febrile infants at low risk for serious bacterial infection—an appraisal of the Rochester criteria and implications for management. Febrile Infant Collaborative Study Group. *Pediatrics*. 1994 Sep;94(3):390–396.

21. Ferrera PC, Bartfield JM, Snyder HS. Neonatal fever: utility of the Rochester criteria in determining low risk for serious bacterial infections. *Am J Emerg Med*. 1997 May;15(3):299–302.

22. Kadish HA, Loveridge B, Tobey J, Bolte RG, Corneli HM. Applying outpatient protocols in febrile infants 1–28 days of age: can the threshold be lowered? *Clin Pediatr*. 2000 Feb;39(2):81–88.

23. Jaye DL, Waites KB. Clinical applications of C-reactive protein in pediatrics. *Pediatr Infect Dis J*. 1997 Aug;16(8):735–746.

24. Ainbender E, Cabatu EE, Guzman DM, Sweet AY. Serum C-reactive protein and problems of newborn infants. *J Pediatr*. 1982 Sep;101(3):438–440.

25. Stein M, Schacter-Davidoff A, Babai I, Tasher D, Somekh E. The accuracy of C-reactive protein, procalcitonin, and s-TREM-1 in the prediction of serious bacterial infection in neonates. *Clin Pediatr*. 2015 May;54(5):439–444.

26. Bilavesky E, Yarden-Bilavesky H, Ashkenazi S, Amir J. C-reactive protein as a marker of serious bacterial infections in hospitalized febrile infants. *Acta Paediatr*. 2009 Nov;98(11):1776–1780.

27. Lacour AG, Zamora SA, Gervaix A. A score identifying serious bacterial infections in children with fever without source. *Pediatr Infect Dis J*. 2008;27:654–656.

28. Galetto-Lacour A, Zamora SA, Andreola B, et al. Validation of a laboratory risk index score for the identification of severe bacterial infection in children with fever without source. *Arch Dis Child*. 2010;95:968–973.

29. Bressan S, Gomez B, Mintegi S, et al. Diagnostic performance of the lab-score in predicting severe and invasive bacterial infections in well-appearing young febrile infants. *Pediatr Infect Dis J*. 2012;31:1239–1244.

30. Gomez B, Mintegi S, Bressan S, et al. Validation of the "step-by-step" approach in the management of young febrile infants. *Pediatrics*. 2016;138. doi:10.1542/peds.2015–4381

31. Mintegi S, Bressan S, Gomez B, et al. Accuracy of a sequential approach to identify young febrile infants at low risk for invasive bacterial infection. *Emerg Med J*. 2014;31(e1):e19–e24.

32. Schwartz S, Raveh D, Toker O, Segal G, Godovitch N, Schlesinger Y. A week-by-week analysis of the low-risk criteria for serious bacterial infection in febrile neonates. *Arch Dis Child*. 2009;94(4):287–292.

33. Simon AE, Lukacs SL, Mendola P. Emergency department laboratory evaluations of fever without source in children aged 3 to 36 months. *Pediatrics*. 2011 Dec;128(6):e1368–e1375.

34. American College of Emergency Physicians Clinical Policies Subcommittee (Writing Committee) on Pediatric Fever, Mace SE, Gemme SR, Valente JH, Eskin

B, Bakes K, Brecher D, Brown MD. Clinical policy for well-appearing infants and children younger than 2 years of age presenting to the emergency department with fever. *Ann Emerg Med*. 2016 May;67(5):625–639.e13.

35. Baraff LJ. Management of infants and young children with fever without source. *Pediatr Ann*. 2008;37(10):673–679.

36. American Academy of Pediatrics, Subcommittee on Urinary Tract Infection, Steering Committee on Quality Improvement and Management. Urinary tract infection: clinical practice guideline for the diagnosis and management of the initial UTI in febrile infants and children 2 to 24 months. *Pediatrics*. 2011;128(3):595–610.

37. Maniaci V, Dauber A, Weiss S, et al. Procalcitonin in young febrile infants for the detection of serious bacterial infections. *Pediatrics*. 2008;122:701–710.

38. Mahajan P, Grzybowski M, Chen X, et al. Procalcitonin as a marker of serious bacterial infections in febrile children younger than 3 years old. *Acad Emerg Med*. 2014;21:171–179.

39. Milcent K, Faesch S, Gras-Le Guen C, et al. Use of procalcitonin assays to predict serious bacterial infection in young febrile infants. *JAMA Pediatr*. 2016;170:62–69.

40. Gomez B, Bressan S, Mintegi S, et al. Diagnostic value of procalcitonin in well-appearing young febrile infants. *Pediatrics*. 2012;130(5):815–822.

41. Woelker JU, Sinha M, Christopher NC, et al. Serum procalcitonin concentration in the evaluation of febrile infants 2 to 60 days of age. *Pediatr Emerg Care*. 2012;28:410–415.

42. Andreola B, Bressan S, Callegaro S, Liverani A, Plebani M, Da Dalt L. Procalcitonin and C-reactive protein as diagnostic markers of severe bacterial infections in febrile infants and children in the emergency department. *Pediatr Infect Dis J*. 2007;26(8):672–677.

43. Yo CH, Hsieh PS, Lee SH, et al. Comparison of the test characteristics of procalcitonin to C-reactive protein and leukocytosis for the detection of serious bacterial infections in children presenting with fever without source: a systematic review and meta-analysis. *Ann Emerg Med*. 2012;60:591–600.

44. Woll C, Neuman MI, Aronson PL. Management of the febrile young infant: update for the 21st century. *Pediatr Emerg Care*. 2017 Nov;33(11):748–753.

45. Hamilton JL, John SP. Evaluation of fever in infants and young children. *Am Fam Physician*. 2013 Feb 15;87(4):254–260.

46. Lee GM, Fleisher GR, Harper MB. Management of febrile children in the age of the conjugate pneumococcal vaccine: a cost-effectiveness analysis. *Pediatrics*. 2001 Oct;108(4):835–844.

47. Jhaveri R, Byington CL, Klein JO, Shapiro ED. Management of the non-toxic-appearing acutely febrile child: a 21st century approach. *J Pediatr*. 2011 Aug;159(2):181–185.

48. Still ML, Rubin LG. Incidence of occult bacteremia among highly febrile young children in the era of the pneumococcal conjugate vaccine: a study from a

Children's Hospital Emergency Department and Urgent Care Center. *Arch Pediatr Adolesc Med*. 2004 Jul;158(7):671–675.

49. Carstairs KL, Tanen DA, Johnson AS, Kailes SB, Riffenburgh RH. Pneumococcal bacteremia in febrile infants presenting to the emergency department before and after the introduction of the heptavalent pneumococcal vaccine. *Ann Emerg Med*. 2007 Jun;49(6):772–777.
50. Sard B, Bailey MC, Vinci R. An analysis of pediatric blood cultures in the postpneumococcal conjugate vaccine era in a community hospital emergency department. *Pediatr Emerg Care*. 2006 May;22(5):295–300.
51. Waddle E, Jhaveri R. Outcomes of febrile children without localising signs after pneumococcal conjugate vaccine. *Arch Dis Child*. 2009 Feb;94(2):144–147.

8 Sepsis Alert

Sriram Ramgopal

A previously healthy 4-year-old girl presents to the emergency department (ED) with complaints of fever and difficulty breathing. She is fully immunized for age. In the ED, she has a temperature of 39.4°C, heart rate of 196 beats per minute, blood pressure of 107/53 mmHg, and a respiratory rate of 38 breaths per minute. Her oxygen saturation is 74%, which promptly increases to 93% on a nonrebreather mask. She is lethargic and has significant tachypnea with accessory muscle use. Her capillary refill time is 4 to 5 seconds. She is given two 20 mL per kilogram boluses of normal saline. Her white blood cell count and absolute neutrophil counts are undetectably low. A chest radiograph is concerning for a right-sided infiltrate, for which she is given cefepime and vancomycin. Even after provision of bolus fluids, antipyretics, and antibiotics, she has a heart rate of 160 beats per minute and a prolonged capillary refill time.

What do you do now?

DISCUSSION

The young girl in this vignette presents with evidence of hemodynamic instability (tachycardia with prolonged capillary refill) despite initial fluid resuscitation. Given her concerning physical examination findings in the setting of a likely infectious (i.e., pulmonary) source, she meets criteria for sepsis. Because she has evidence of cardiovascular organ dysfunction, she also meets criteria for septic shock. Between 20,000 to 40,000 children in the United States develop severe sepsis annually with a mortality rate of 5% to 10%. In one multicenter, international study, approximately 20% of survivors have at least moderate disability as a sequela of their illness. The prevalence of sepsis diagnosed in U.S. children's hospitals may be increasing, though with a gradually decreasing rate of mortality.

The diagnostic criteria for pediatric sepsis was published in 2005 by the International Consensus Conference on Pediatric Sepsis and is based on the definition of systemic inflammatory response syndrome (SIRS). To have SIRS, a patient must meet two of the following criteria: (1) fever (≥38.5°C) or hypothermia (<36°C), (2) tachycardia over 2 standard deviations for age or bradycardia in an infant, (3) tachypnea over 2 standard deviations for age or mechanical ventilation in a patient not given general anesthesia and without underlying neuromuscular disease, and (4) elevated or depressed leukocyte count or >10% immature neutrophils. The term *sepsis* is applied when an infection is suspected to be the cause of SIRS. *Severe sepsis* is characterized by sepsis with cardiovascular organ dysfunction, acute respiratory distress syndrome, or dysfunction of two or more organ systems (respiratory, neurologic, hematologic, renal, or hepatic). *Septic shock* is when sepsis is complicated by cardiovascular organ dysfunction. Given the remarkable physiologic reserve of children, hypotension lacks sensitivity for serious illness and is considered a late finding in pediatric septic shock, as children preserve cardiac output by increasing heart rate and systemic vascular resistance. Evidence of cardiovascular organ dysfunction may instead be appreciated by the presence of unexplained metabolic acidosis, elevated lactate, oliguria, prolonged capillary refill, or a difference in core to peripheral temperature by 3°C.

Several difficulties with this definition have been identified. First, the reliance on vital signs and complete blood count parameters in pediatric

SIRS criteria requires familiarity with the use of age-specific normative values. Second, children often demonstrate wide changes in vital signs in response to a variety of more benign conditions, such as viral illnesses, asthma exacerbations, or bronchiolitis. Heart rate and respiratory rate both rise in the setting of fever from any source. Approximately 15% of children present to the ED with a fever, for example, and of these, greater than 90% demonstrate SIRS vital signs. Third, there is poor concordance between patients diagnosed with sepsis by physicians to those meeting the formal definition, with physicians diagnosing severe sepsis more broadly. As a result, it may be difficult to translate findings from research into clinical practice.

The terms "warm" and "cold" shock are frequently used to describe distinct pathophysiologic states. In adults, septic shock presents more commonly as a form of distributive or warm shock, characterized by wide pulse pressure (in which the diastolic blood pressure is less than one half of the systolic blood pressure), brisk capillary refill, and warm extremities. Cold shock is manifested as a narrow pulse pressure, suggestive of a low stroke volume or high systemic vascular resistance, prolonged capillary refill, and cold extremities. Patients with warm shock are more fluid resistant compared to those with cold shock. Clinical differentiation between these presentations of shock in children is prone to error. In one prospective evaluation of hemodynamics of pediatric patients presenting with sepsis, those with an indwelling central line were more likely to have warm shock, whereas those with community-acquired sepsis were more likely to have cold shock.

The critical aspect of management of sepsis lies in prompt recognition of potential cases. Delayed recognition and treatment of shock is associated with an increasing risk of poor outcomes, including death. In one study, each delayed hour of treatment for pediatric sepsis was associated with greater than a two-fold increased odds of mortality. Sepsis can present in previously healthy patients, but approximately 70% of cases of sepsis occur in those with an underlying complex condition. High-risk factors include chronic neuromuscular conditions, immunocompromise, transplant, asplenia (including functional asplenia, as in patients with sickle cell disease), presence of central line, or malignancy. Salient physical exam findings include a prolonged or "flashy" capillary refill, decreased or bounding pulse, mottled skin or skin with petechiae, alterations in mental status (evidence of cerebral hypoperfusion), hepatomegaly, and pulmonary rales.

Given the limited ability to identify sepsis on the basis of vital signs or physical examination, the use of biomarkers has long been an area of active interest. Unfortunately, there is no single diagnostic test to reliably identify cases of sepsis in children. Lactic acid measurements are frequently used in adults, but because children clear lactic acid more quickly, measurement of this biomarker is not a reliable diagnostic test. However, lactic acid may be indicative of early organ dysfunction and correlates with 30-day mortality. A single measurement of C-reactive protein has poor diagnostic accuracy for pediatric sepsis, though serial measurements may be of value. Procalcitonin may have improved diagnostic value compared to C-reactive protein, particularly early in the course of evaluation. For the clinician in the ED, the diagnosis of sepsis will ultimately rely on a suspicion based on vital signs, supplemented by laboratory testing, with a tolerance of uncertainty in most cases.

Once sepsis is identified, treatment should be prompt (Figure 8.1). Supplemental oxygen should be provided. If available central lines should be accessed and an additional peripheral line should be obtained. The use of ultrasonography may be helpful in patients with difficult access. If these measures are unsuccessful, an intraosseous line should be placed. Diagnostic studies should include blood cultures from all central lines (if applicable) in addition to a peripheral culture, urine cultures, and respiratory cultures in patients who are intubated or with a tracheostomy. Though cultures are ideal, treatment should not be delayed if they cannot be readily acquired. Additional diagnostic tests include complete blood cell counts, urinalysis, cortisol level, chest radiography, and blood gas measurement. Empiric broad-spectrum antimicrobial therapy should be initiated. Bolus fluids in 20 mL per kilogram alloquats have proven benefit in patients with sepsis. Boluses should be administered over 5 to 10 minutes. This can be facilitated by the use of the push-pull technique or with a pressure bag but not with gravity techniques (Figure 8.2a and 8.2b). Up to 60 mL per kilogram can be provided in the first hour, unless hepatomegaly or rales develop. Therapeutic endpoints should include a capillary refill ≤2 seconds, normal blood pressure for age, normal pulses, urine output >1 mL per kilogram per hour, and normal mental status.

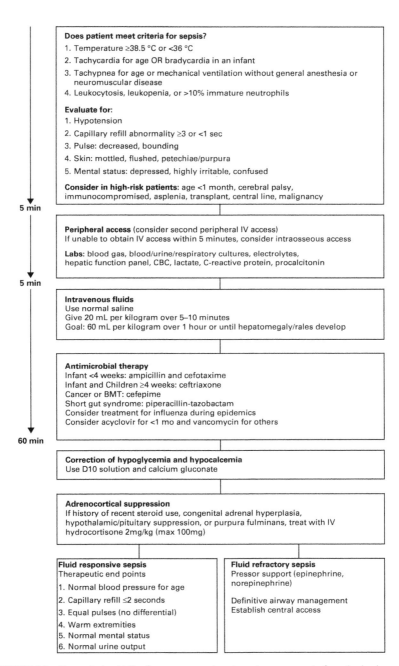

5 min

Does patient meet criteria for sepsis?
1. Temperature ≥38.5 °C or <36 °C
2. Tachycardia for age OR bradycardia in an infant
3. Tachypnea for age or mechanical ventilation without general anesthesia or neuromuscular disease
4. Leukocytosis, leukopenia, or >10% immature neutrophils

Evaluate for:
1. Hypotension
2. Capillary refill abnormality ≥3 or <1 sec
3. Pulse: decreased, bounding
4. Skin: mottled, flushed, petechiae/purpura
5. Mental status: depressed, highly irritable, confused

Consider in high-risk patients: age <1 month, cerebral palsy, immunocompromised, asplenia, transplant, central line, malignancy

5 min

Peripheral access (consider second peripheral IV access)
If unable to obtain IV access within 5 minutes, consider intraosseous access

Labs: blood gas, blood/urine/respiratory cultures, electrolytes, hepatic function panel, CBC, lactate, C-reactive protein, procalcitonin

Intravenous fluids
Use normal saline
Give 20 mL per kilogram over 5–10 minutes
Goal: 60 mL per kilogram over 1 hour or until hepatomegaly/rales develop

60 min

Antimicrobial therapy
Infant <4 weeks: ampicillin and cefotaxime
Infant and Children ≥4 weeks: ceftriaxone
Cancer or BMT: cefepime
Short gut syndrome: piperacillin-tazobactam
Consider treatment for influenza during epidemics
Consider acyclovir for <1 mo and vancomycin for others

Correction of hypoglycemia and hypocalcemia
Use D10 solution and calcium gluconate

Adrenocortical suppression
If history of recent steroid use, congenital adrenal hyperplasia, hypothalamic/pituitary suppression, or purpura fulminans, treat with IV hydrocortisone 2mg/kg (max 100mg)

Fluid responsive sepsis
Therapeutic end points
1. Normal blood pressure for age
2. Capillary refill ≤2 seconds
3. Equal pulses (no differential)
4. Warm extremities
5. Normal mental status
6. Normal urine output

Fluid refractory sepsis
Pressor support (epinephrine, norepinephrine)

Definitive airway management
Establish central access

FIGURE 8.1. Suggested guideline for emergency department management of septic shock. MV, mechanical ventilation; GA, general anesthesia; IV, intravenous; CBC, complete blood count with differential.

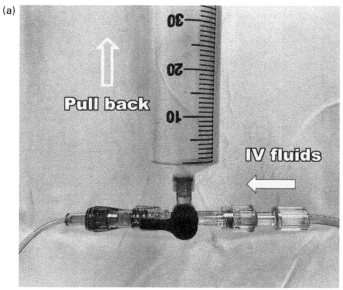

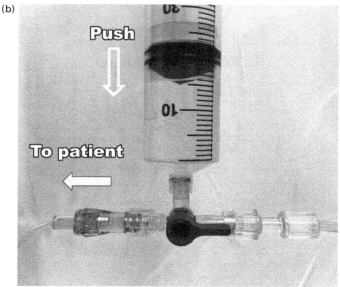

FIGURE 8.2. Push-pull system for rapid bolus of intravenous fluids: (a) A three-way stopcock is initially off to the patient and intravenous fluids are pulled into a large 60 mL syringe from the intravenous fluid bag, then (b) the stopcock is placed off to the bag so that the fluid in the syringe can be rapidly pushed toward the patient.

The choice of antibiotic to use in sepsis should be broad spectrum and should be tailored to patient risk factors and local epidemiology. Pneumococcal sepsis is increasingly rare following immunization measures, but isolates of pneumococcus have a higher rate of antimicrobial resistance. Patients with neutropenia should receive antipseudomonal coverage. Coverage for methicillin-resistance staphylococcus aureus should be provided in endemic regions. Clindamyin, an inhibitor of protein synthesis, may be considered as an additional therapy in cases of toxic shock syndrome. Empiric treatment for influenza should be initiated if the patient presents during an epidemic.

Fluid refractory shock is defined as shock in which perfusion fails to improve after provision of at least 60 mL per kilogram of bolused fluids or if the development hepatomegaly and rales preclude further boluses. Pressors should be used in such cases. Epinephrine is a beta and alpha agonist with positive inotropic and chronotropic effects. It does not aggravate vasoconstriction at lower doses and is therefore ideal for cold shock. Norepinephrine is an alpha agonist that primarily has a vasoconstrictive effect and is therefore better suited for warm shock. While the subject of some debate, extrapolated data from adults suggest that even norepinephrine can be given peripherally for a short period of approximately 4 hours through a large bore intravenous (IV) 18- or 20-gauge needle placed at a level at or above the antecubital fossa. A dilute concentration of pressor should be used when given peripherally. Pressors should be titrated to adequate blood pressure and perfusion. Though dopamine is recommended as an alternative to epinephrine in cold shock in "Surviving Sepsis" guidelines, it is rarely used. In addition to pressor support, patients with fluid refractory and catecholamine resistant shock with a known or suspected adrenal insufficiency should be given IV hydrocortisone.

Endotracheal intubation may be required for patients with shock because of underlying respiratory disease or disordered control of breathing. Cardiovascular instability is less likely to occur if adequate fluid resuscitation has been performed prior to intubation. Pediatric patients with sepsis have a higher rate of complications following intubation compared to nonelective intubation performed for other indications, with hypotension being the most common serious adverse event. Ketamine, which usually causes tachycardia and hypertension and does not compromise respiratory drive, may be better suited for sedation or rapid sequence intubation, though it carries risk of peri-intubation vomiting. While still likely the safest drug for rapid sequence intubation for most patients, studies in adults suggest that ketamine can cause delayed hypotension in some patients with a shock index (pulse rate divided by systolic blood pressure) greater than 0.9. Etomidate is an inhibitor of 11β-hydroxylase, an enzyme involved in steroidogenesis. While a single dose of etomidate in a patient without known adrenal insufficiency is unlikely to have significant effects, there is sufficient concern such that expert guidelines do not suggest its use in a septic patient. Propofol is a powerful myocardial depressant and should be avoided to prevent worsening of hypotension.

Given the rarity of sepsis and the prevalence of SIRS-consistent vital signs in the ED and the association of early treatment with better outcomes, a large focus of research has searched for ways to identify sepsis early in the ED setting. One such mechanism lies in the use of trigger tools built into electronic medical record systems to identify candidate cases, typically based on vital signs. These trigger tools can then be paired with "packages," or action plans consisting of blood cultures, bolus fluids, and IV antibiotics. The mandated institution of a package in the state of New York, for example, where patients with suspected sepsis were required to receive a blood culture, antibiotics, and 20 mL per kilogram bolus within 1 hour of presentation, resulted in improved outcomes for those receiving care according to benchmarks. However, these guidelines are still not widespread in a large number of adult and pediatric centers in the United States, demonstrating important gaps in care. Additionally, these trigger tools carry the risk of alarm burnout, given their high sensitivity but poor specificity.

For the patient in this vignette, her perfusion failed to improve and she was placed on pressor support. Because of declining mental status and respiratory failure, she was emergently intubated following admission to the pediatric intensive care unit and ultimately required veno-arterial extracorporeal membrane oxygenation for greater than 1 month. During admission, infectious testing was only positive for influenza. Despite a course complicated by renal, hematologic, and hepatic dysfunction, she exhibited excellent neurologic recovery.

Pediatric sepsis remains a complex disease with a high morbidity and mortality. For the ED provider, the primary challenge in sepsis lies in prompt recognition of potential cases and providing resuscitation, with an appreciation for the uncertainty in many cases early in disease presentation. The mainstays of ED therapy are fluid resuscitation with empiric antimicrobial coverage, ideally within the first hour of presentation.

KEY POINTS

- Pediatric sepsis is defined as the presence of SIRS (fever/hypothermia, tachycardia, tachypnea, and leukopenia/leukocytosis) in a patient with a presumed infectious etiology; septic shock is sepsis in the presence of cardiovascular organ dysfunction.
- Hypotension is a late finding in pediatric sepsis.
- Early treatment with intravascular resuscitation and antibiotics, ideally within 60 minutes of presentation, is associated with improved outcomes in pediatric sepsis.

Further Reading

Balamuth F, Weiss SL, Neuman MI, et al. Pediatric severe sepsis in U.S. children's hospitals. *Pediatr Crit Care Med.* 2014;15(9):798–805. doi:10.1097/PCC.0000000000000225

Brierley J, Peters MJ. Distinct hemodynamic patterns of septic shock at presentation to pediatric intensive care. *Pediatrics.* 2008;122(4):752–759. doi:10.1542/peds.2007-1979

Carcillo JA, Davis AL, Zaritsky A. Role of early fluid resuscitation in pediatric septic shock. *JAMA.* 1991;266(9):1242–1245. http://www.ncbi.nlm.nih.gov/pubmed/1870250

Dellinger RP, Levy MM, Rhodes A, et al. Surviving Sepsis campaign: international guidelines for management of severe sepsis and septic shock, 2012. *Intensive Care Med.* 2013;39(2):165–228. doi:10.1007/s00134-012-2769-8

Evans IVR, Phillips GS, Alpern ER, et al. Association between the New York sepsis care mandate and in-hospital mortality for pediatric sepsis. *JAMA.* 2018;320(4):358. doi:10.1001/jama.2018.9071

Goldstein B, Giroir B, Randolph A, International Consensus Conference on Pediatric Sepsis. International Pediatric Sepsis Consensus Conference: definitions for sepsis and organ dysfunction in pediatrics. *Pediatr Crit Care Med*. 2005;6(1):2–8. doi:10.1097/01.PCC.0000149131.72248.E6

Han YY, Carcillo JA, Dragotta MA, et al. Early reversal of pediatric-neonatal septic shock by community physicians is associated with improved outcome. *Pediatrics*. 2003;112(4):793–799. http://www.ncbi.nlm.nih.gov/pubmed/14523168

Miller M, Kruit N, Heldreich C, et al. Hemodynamic response after rapid sequence induction with ketamine in out-of-hospital patients at risk of shock as defined by the Shock Index. *Ann Emerg Med*. 2016;68(2):181–188.e2. doi:10.1016/j.annemergmed.2016.03.041

Odetola FO, Gebremariam A, Freed GL. Patient and hospital correlates of clinical outcomes and resource utilization in severe pediatric sepsis. *Pediatrics*. 2007;119(3):487–494. doi:10.1542/peds.2006-2353

Scott HF, Deakyne SJ, Woods JM, Bajaj L. The prevalence and diagnostic utility of systemic inflammatory response syndrome vital signs in a pediatric emergency department. *Acad Emerg Med*. 2015;22(4):381–389. doi:10.1111/acem.12610

Scott HF, Donoghue AJ, Gaieski DF, Marchese RF, Mistry RD. The utility of early lactate testing in undifferentiated pediatric systemic inflammatory response syndrome. *Acad Emerg Med*. 2012;19(11):1276–1280. doi:10.1111/acem.12014

Weiss SL, Fitzgerald JC, Maffei FA, et al. Discordant identification of pediatric severe sepsis by research and clinical definitions in the SPROUT international point prevalence study. *Crit Care*. 2015;19(1):325. doi:10.1186/s13054-015-1055-x

Weiss SL, Fitzgerald JC, Pappachan J, et al. Global epidemiology of pediatric severe sepsis: the sepsis prevalence, outcomes, and therapies study. *Am J Respir Crit Care Med*. 2015;191(10):1147–1157. doi:10.1164/rccm.201412-2323OC

9 What Goes Down, Might Come Up!

Sharon E. Mace

A 6-month-old male is brought to the emergency department because of non-bilious, non-bloody vomiting. He was well when his mother left for work but when she came home he was vomiting. He is "sleepier" and "less active" than usual and not feeding well. He has had no fever, diarrhea, coughing, or trouble breathing. He has not had any recent illnesses. The household includes the mother and her boyfriend. There are no siblings.

Past medical history is unremarkable. He was the full-term product of uncomplicated pregnancy, labor, and delivery. His birth weight was 7 pounds. His immunizations are up to date. The temperature is 98.6°F, pulse 96 and regular, respirations 24, and oxygen saturation 98% on room air. The lungs, cardiac, abdominal, ENT, and extremity examination is unremarkable. The skin has normal turgor and no rashes, petechiae, or signs of trauma.

What do you do now?

DISCUSSION

The differential diagnosis of vomiting in infants is extensive, but a thorough history and examination can lead to the etiology and appropriate management (Table 9.1). The symptoms and the patient's age generally suggest a diagnosis.

Determine whether the infant has vomiting or is "spitting up." This is important because, although parents are often concerned, the causes of spitting up are rarely serious, while vomiting can be from a life-threatening condition. Spitting up is the *effortless* regurgitation of esophageal or gastric contents and is commonly due to overfeeding or gastroesophageal reflux (GER). Physiologic reflux peaks at 4 months of age and usually resolves by 1 year of age. Infants with *benign* GER, dubbed "happy spitters," have normal growth (including weight gain) and development and do not need acid suppressant therapy. Benign GER should be differentiated from GER disease (GERD), which is characterized by additional symptoms such as poor feeding, weight loss, and irritability.

VOMITING DEFINITION

Vomiting is the *forceful* expulsion of esophageal or gastric contents into the mouth. Vomiting is a protective reflux. The emetic reflux is a mechanism designed to protect the body against intestinal distention, toxins, and other harmful conditions.

CHARACTERISTICS OF THE VOMITING

What about the vomiting? Is it effortless or forceful, projectile or not, bilious or bloody, acute or chronic? Bilious vomiting in an infant usually indicates bowel obstruction and therefore *always* merits emergent evaluation. Bile-colored emesis occurs with reflux of duodenal fluid into the stomach, while gastric fluid is usually yellow-tinged. Bright red blood, especially with the first emesis, suggests active bleeding. Coffee-ground emesis indicates stomach acid has reacted with the blood. Blood occurring after several episodes of vomiting implies a Mallory-Weiss tear. Projectile vomiting in a 1-month-old first-born male suggests pyloric stenosis. What

TABLE 9.1 **Causes of Vomiting: Gastrointestinal and Nongastrointestinal**

Gastrointestinal
Physiologic gastrointestinal reflux
Infant rumination, adolescent rumination
Achalasia
Gastroesophageal reflux disease (GERD)
Gastroenteritis: viral (such as rotavirus)
Gastroenteritis: bacterial (such as salmonella, shigella)
Celiac disease
Colitis

Severe constipation/Obstipation

Necrotizing enterocolitis (NEC)

Inflammatory bowel disease (IBD), Crohn's disease, ulcerative colitis

Diet or formula related: dietary protein intolerance or allergy: milk protein-induced enteritis, food-protein induced enteropathy

Feeding related or intolerance – over-feeding

Associated with systemic disorders: heart failure: tire with feeding, pulmonary/respiratory distress, neuromuscular disorders: lack coordination of muscles needed for feeding

Hepatobiliary disease: hepatitis (see also infection), cholecystitis, congenital: biliary atresia

Obstruction - Congenital: pyloric stenosis, congenital stenosis or atresia or web or stricture, malrotation with mid-gut volvulus, volvulus, intussusception, Hirschsprung disease, annular pancreas, tracheoesophageal fistula

Obstruction- non-congenital: foreign body, bezoar, adhesions, tumor, superior mesenteric artery (SMA) syndrome

Eosinophilic esophagitis/gastroenteritis

Appendicitis
Gastritis
Esophagitis
Ileus
Pancreatitis
Peritonitis
Gastroparesis
Pseudo-obstruction
Cyclical vomiting

TABLE 9.1 **Continued**

Nongastrointestinal

Nongastrointestinal Infections: otitis media, pharyngitis, respiratory tract infections/pneumonia, urinary tract infection/pyelonephritis

Serious infections: bacteremia, sepsis, central nervous system infections: meningitis, encephalitis, brain abscess (see also neurologic)

Neurologic: meningitis, encephalitis, brain abscess, tumor, mass, hydrocephalus, pseudotumor cerebri, increased intracranial pressure (from any cause including shaken baby syndrome), abdominal migraine, migraine

Endocrine: Diabetic ketoacidosis, adrenal insufficiency

Metabolic - Inborn errors of metabolism (IEM): carbohydrate metabolism disorders, galactosemia, hereditary fructose intolerance, organic acidemias, urea cycle disorders

Genitourinary/Renal: urinary tract infection/pyelonephritis, renal stones, obstructive uropathy, renal insufficiency, testicular torsion, epididymitis

Pulmonary/Respiratory: post-tussive emesis

Hepatobiliary disease: liver failure, cholecystitis, biliary atresia

Drugs: prescription, over the counter: acetaminophen, salicylates, chemotherapeutic medications, others

Drugs of abuse: alcohol, THC (cannaboid hyperemesis syndrome)

Toxins: mushroom poisoning, iron, lead

Vestibular: motion sickness, acute labyrinthitis, otitis

Child (physical) maltreatment: duodenal hematoma, pancreatitis, bowel rupture, ruptured liver and/or spleen, etc. (usually presents as acute gastrointestinal disease, shock, etc.), Munchausen syndrome

Obstetric: pregnancy (morning sickness)

Psychiatric: eating disorders – bulimia (binge and purge), psychogenic vomiting, emotional response to strong smell or taste, fear, anger

Other: Reyes syndrome

Hernia – incarcerated hernia

This is not an all-inclusive list but includes most of the common or serious/life-threatening causes of vomiting in the pediatric patient.

Italics represent common and/or serious etiologies for vomiting in infants.

TABLE 9.1 **Continued**

Red Flags: Concerning Signs and Symptoms in the Vomiting Infant

History: Symptoms

Altered mental status such as lethargy, listlessness, unresponsiveness signifies serious, usually life-threatening disease

Bilious vomiting suggests intestinal obstruction especially in an infant

Projectile vomiting: consider pyloric stenosis especially in a first-born male infant 6 weeks to 6 months of age

Periodic vomiting: consider inborn error of metabolism especially in absence of signs of obstruction (no abdominal distention, no abdominal tenderness on palpation, may have unusual odor and/or cataracts)

Prolonged vomiting: > 12 hours in neonate, > 24 hours in infant (1 month up to 24 months), > 48 hours in older child

Bloody vomiting (hematemesis) or coffee ground emesis indicates GI bleeding

Diarrhea especially with blood in the stool: bacterial gastroenteritis, IBD, Hirschprung's disease, necrotizing enterocolitis, colitis from multiple etiologies

Rectal bleeding especially "current jelly" stool suggests intussusception in an infant

Recurrent infections (e.g. pneumonia) and vomiting raises concern for TEF

Headache and vomiting are suggestive of a CNS etiology for the vomiting

Vital Signs and weight

Fever may be associated with viral gastroenteritis but may also be associated with NEC, IBD, appendicitis, etc. and infections

Abnormal vital signs: fever or hypothermia can be associated with infections, tachycardia may be present with dehydration, tachypnea can occur with serious infection or a respiratory illness or be compensation for a metabolic acidosis (inborn error of metabolism) or Kussmaul respirations with DKA, and low blood pressure or shock suggests life threatening infection (such as sepsis) or severe dehydration or both

Weight

Poor weight gain or failure to thrive always needs evaluation

Physical Examination

Abdominal examination

Abdominal distention generally indicates obstruction, ileus, or ascites

Abnormal bowel sounds: absent bowel sounds or high-pitched bowel sounds – "borborygimi" signifies obstruction

TABLE 9.1 **Continued**

Jaundice signifies hepatobiliary disease

Organomegaly: hepatomegaly can occur with liver disease or IEM, splenomegaly can occur with metabolic disorders

Focal abdominal tenderness can suggest an etiology for the vomiting: RLQ pain – appendicitis; RUQ pain – hepatobiliary disease; LLQ pain-colitis.

While perhaps not immediately life-threatening, other focal abdominal tenderness raises consideration for a possible etiology for the vomiting: epigastric tenderness – gastritis, esophagitis, pancreatitis; suprapubic tenderness – UTI, flank tenderness – pyelonephritis

Neurologic examination: Findings (eg., focal neurologic findings, bulging fontanelle, stiff neck) mandates a thorough neurologic exam and evaluation for increased intracranial pressure, physical child maltreatment (shaken baby syndrome), hydrocephalus, CNS infections (meningitis, encephalitis, brain abscess)

Ataxia can occur with CNS disease or vestibular disorders

Other Examination

Skin examination: check for bruises, unusual marks or burns as with physical abuse as well as for other clues - color: pale, cyanotic, jaundice; severe dehydration or shock: diaphoretic, poor turgor, delayed capillary fill; for infection: rash, petechiae; and for bleeding disorders: purpura,

Cardiovascular: remember heart failure can be a cause of poor feeding/ vomiting

Genitourinary Examination: rule out congenital adrenal hyperplasia in an infant with ambiguous genitalia with vomiting (and hyperkalemia); check males for testicular torsion and check for incarcerated hernias

HEENT: look in the mouth/throat for pharyngitis or stomatitis, the ears for otitis

Head/neck: consider life-threatening infections: check for a bulging fontanelle that occurs with increased intracranial pressure, consider intracranial injury with signs of head and/or facial trauma, check for neck stiffness with meningitis

Respiratory: listen to the lungs for rales with pneumonia

Abnormal smell or odor can be suggestive of IEM such as maple syrup urine disease

Other "pearls"

Always consider non-GI in addition to GI disorders.

Infection, congenital diseases, and child maltreatment are in the differential about the duration of vomiting? Prolonged vomiting is suggestive of a serious etiology such as obstruction. The definition of prolonged vomiting varies according to age: neonates >12 hours, infants >24 hours, and >48 hours in older children.

Are there recurrent episodes of vomiting? In an infant with recurrent vomiting and a benign abdominal exam, inborn errors of metabolism or new onset diabetic ketoacidosis are in the differential. Is the vomiting acute, chronic, or cyclic? In the infant, acute, episodic vomiting can occur with intestinal malrotation with intermittent volvulus, inborn errors of metabolism, and food-protein-induced enterocolitis syndrome. Chronic vomiting can occur with adverse reactions to food or eosinophilic esophagitis and, generally in older patients, gall bladder disease or peptic ulcer disease. With cyclical vomiting syndrome, which usually occurs at an older age, episodes of vomiting are interspersed with symptom-free periods of no vomiting.

RELATIONSHIP OF VOMITING TO FEEDING

How often and how much is the infant feeding? Infants have a limited gastric capacity. Is the parent giving too much formula at one time and overfeeding the infant, instead of giving smaller amounts of formula more frequently?

Is there a temporal relationship of the feeding to the vomiting? Vomiting immediately after eating implies an esophageal etiology, particularly if the emesis contains undigested food, as may occur with achalasia or eosinophilic esophagitis. Emesis occurring minutes to hours after feeding implies a gastric source as with gastroparesis. Vomiting that occurs after fasting is typical of inborn errors of metabolism.

FORMULA OR DIET

What about the diet or formula? Consider an inborn error of metabolism if there is vomiting after a large protein meal or biliary disease if there is vomiting after ingestion of fatty foods as occurs with cholecystitis. Vomiting after a feeding of cow's milk may be indicative of a cow's milk intolerance or allergy, and a change in formula may eliminate the vomiting. Food protein induced enterocolitis is characterized by acute episodic vomiting after the ingestion of protein.

ASSOCIATED SYMPTOMS

Abdominal Pain

Are there associated symptoms? Is there abdominal pain, or is it painless vomiting? Most surgical emergencies, such as obstruction, are associated with pain. Is the infant lying with his or her legs drawn up in order to alleviate the pain? Is the infant crying or irritable? Does palpation of the abdomen precipitate crying, or does the older child try to pull away or push the examiner's hand away? The location of the pain is valuable information. Localization of the pain to the right lower quadrant could be appendicitis, while right upper quadrant tenderness on palpation can occur with hepatitis or hepatobiliary disease including cholecystitis. Epigastric tenderness is typically found with gastritis, peptic ulcer disease, pancreatitis, or a duodenal hematoma (as with child physical maltreatment). Suprapubic tenderness may be seen with urinary tract infections, and flank pain may be present with pyelonephritis or other kidney diseases. Lower abdominal pain is typical of inflammatory bowel disease or constipation.

Diarrhea

Are there other gastrointestinal (GI) symptoms? Is diarrhea present? The combination of non-bilious, non-projectile vomiting and non-bloody, non-mucousy diarrhea in an afebrile infant or an infant with a low-grade fever and sick contacts suggests viral gastroenteritis such as rotavirus, while bacterial gastroenteritis is often associated with a higher fever and bloody (e.g., Salmonella) or profuse watery (e.g., Shigella) diarrhea.

Other Associated Symptoms

Does the emesis occur after a severe episode of coughing, as with post-tussive emesis due to increased abdominal pressure? Is there a fever that suggests an infection? Is diarrhea also present, and what are the characteristics of the diarrhea (loose, watery, mucousy, bloody)? Since infections, ranging from pharyngitis, otitis, pneumonia, urinary tract infection, and even sepsis, can cause vomiting, does the infant have symptoms or signs of an infection elsewhere? Look for any evidence of any central nervous system illness/injury since increased intracranial pressure can lead to vomiting.

PAST MEDICAL HISTORY

Past medical history (PMH) should include neonatal history, growth and development, and social and family history. Was this infant the product of a normal pregnancy, labor, and delivery with a normal birth weight? Were there any problems in the newborn period? Are the immunizations up to date? Has the growth and development been normal? Has the infant been gaining weight? Are there any medical problems in the family? What is the household like? Who cares for the infant? Are there siblings, and are they well with no medical illnesses? Any sick contacts? Recent travel or well water? Any medical problems or surgeries? Is the poor weight gain consistent with failure to thrive? Is there a familial or genetic disorder in the family?

PHYSICAL EXAMINATION

What is the general appearance of the infant? Is he or she toxic, lethargic, or irritable with unstable vital signs or generally well appearing? Is there an unusual appearance of the child, as with a syndrome? Note whether the head is normocephalic and atraumatic. Is the fontanelle full (suggesting increased intracranial pressure) or sunken (indicating dehydration)? Are the eyes sunken, indicating dehydration, or jaundiced, indicating hepatobiliary disease? If the infant cries, are tears present or absent, signifying dehydration? The ears should be examined for otitis media. Note whether there is pharyngitis or stomatitis and if the mucous membranes are moist or dry, indicative of dehydration. Look for adenopathy, swelling, or masses in the neck and check if the neck is supple. Listen to the lungs (rales suggest pneumonia or failure, wheezing suggests bronchiolitis or asthma). Note any respiratory distress or tachypnea. Is there tachypnea, which may be secondary to a respiratory infection such as pneumonia or respiratory compensation for a metabolic acidosis? Is the cardiac exam normal? Is there tachycardia present and if so, is it from dehydration, infection, or pain? Are the extremities normal? The skin turgor should be noted and the skin checked for rashes, petechiae, and trauma. On the abdominal exam, is there distention, tenderness on palpation, any masses ("olive" with pyloric stenosis), or abnormal bowel sounds (hyperactive, tympanitic)? Are there stigmata of a syndrome or chromosomal abnormality? For example, Down syndrome is associated with intestinal atresia.

MANAGEMENT

Vomiting can lead to dehydration, electrolyte abnormalities, and even hypovolemic shock. Aspiration pneumonia is another less common complication of vomiting. Therefore, resuscitation and attention to the ABCs (airway, breathing, and circulation) is the first order of business. Replace fluids and correct electrolyte abnormalities. If dehydration is mild, then oral rehydration may be possible. Ondansetron may be administered for the vomiting. Treat any underlying disorders or injuries that may be causing the vomiting.

In our case study, you obtain further history and reexamine the infant. You order electrolytes, blood urea nitrogen, creatinine, complete blood count, and urinalysis. They are normal.

There has been no dietary changes and the vomiting is not associated with feeding. His growth and development and weight gain have been normal. There have been no prior episodes of vomiting. The emesis is non-bilious and non-bloody. The stool in the diaper is normal (no blood or diarrhea). Family history is negative. Social history reveals the mother left the child in the care of her boyfriend who is not the infant's father. There has been no fever or symptoms/signs of infection. The child has no abnormal facies or stigmata of any syndrome. The abdominal exam is normal with no tenderness, no distention, and normal bowel sounds; the skin is normal. The fontanelle is now full and bulging.

There are several "red flags." The infant has had acute vomiting for over 12 hours and is lethargic. The benign abdominal exam mitigates against obstruction or other GI disorders. History and exam go against infection. Metabolic disorders are unlikely due to normal laboratory studies. You order a computer tomography brain scan, which reveals a central nervous system bleed. A neurosurgery consult is obtained. The infant is admitted to the pediatric intensive care unit where an ophthalmology consult is obtained and confirms hemorrhages consistent with the diagnosis of shaken baby syndrome. The boyfriend later confesses to shaking the infant because he was crying.

KEY POINTS

- Vomiting is usually benign but can portend significant underlying illness or injury.
- Vomiting can be from the GI tract itself but can also be due to more generalized, systemic disorders or injuries (non-GI causes).
- The past medical history in infants includes neonatal history, growth, and developmental history (include weight gain), social history, and family history.
- Bilious vomiting in an infant occurs with obstruction; therefore, bilious vomiting always warrants evaluation.

Further Reading

Florez ID, Niño-Serna LF, Beltrán-Arroyave CP. Acute infectious diarrhea and gastroenteritis in children. *Curr Infect Dis Rep.* 2020 Jan;22(2):4. doi:10.1007/s11908-020-0713-6. Review. PMID: 31993758.

Shields, TM, Lightdale, JR. Vomiting in children. *Pediat Rev.* 2018 Jul; 39(7):342–358. doi:https://doi.org/10.1542/pir.2017-0053

Singhi SC1, Shah R, Bansal A, Jayashree M. Management of a child with vomiting. *Indian J Pediatr.* 2013 Apr;80(4):318–325. doi:10.1007/s12098-012-0959-6. Epub 2013 Jan 23.

10 Was It Something I Ate?

Maytal Firnberg, Laurie Malia, and Joni E. Rabiner

A previously healthy 12-year-old male presents to the emergency department with the onset of sharp abdominal pain today. He ate pizza at school for lunch, and then he started feeling periumbilical abdominal pain that increased throughout the day. He left soccer practice early because running worsened his abdominal pain. This evening, his pain became more severe and right-sided; he refused dinner and began to feel nauseous. Mom brought him to the emergency department where he vomited once. At triage, his vital signs were temperature 101°F orally, heart rate 112 beats per minute, respiratory rate 18 breaths per minute, blood pressure 104/72, and oxygen saturation 100% on room air. His pain is rated as 8/10 in severity. On physical examination, he is in moderate distress secondary to abdominal pain. His abdominal exam is significant for tenderness to palpation localized to the right lower quadrant (RLQ) with rebound tenderness elicited when releasing pressure from the left lower quadrant and voluntary guarding. His genitourinary exam is normal.

What do you do now?

DISCUSSION

In this child with acute onset periumbilical abdominal pain that migrates to the RLQ associated with fever, nausea, and vomiting, appendicitis is high on the differential diagnosis and is a diagnosis not to be missed. However, many other conditions may present with similar signs and symptoms, requiring the clinician to maintain a wide differential diagnosis when evaluating a patient with abdominal pain. Gastroenteritis, constipation, intestinal obstruction, urinary tract infection, ovarian or testicular torsion, intussusception, mesenteric adenitis, and ectopic pregnancy are just some of the pathologies that can also present with abdominal pain. A combination of history, physical exam findings, laboratory results, and imaging is used to differentiate acute appendicitis from other causes of abdominal pain.

Appendicitis is infection or inflammation of the appendix, a tube-like structure attached to the cecum, usually due to luminal obstruction of the appendix. It is the most common indication for emergency abdominal surgery in childhood. Despite its frequency, the diagnosis of appendicitis remains a challenge as history and physical examination findings have variable accuracy and clinical scoring systems such as the Pediatric Appendicitis Score and Alvarado Score have not been shown to be sufficiently reliable, with sensitivity and specificity less than 85%.[1] Furthermore, timely diagnosis and subsequent intervention are essential in acute appendicitis as, without treatment, luminal obstruction may progress to appendiceal perforation, which leads to increased morbidity. As such, it is important for the clinician to recognize the clinical manifestations, understand the utility of laboratory testing, and appreciate when and how to image children who present with acute onset abdominal pain concerning for appendicitis.

The classic presentation of appendicitis begins with the acute onset of periumbilical abdominal pain that migrates to the RLQ within hours. Pain often worsens over time as the disease progresses and increases with walking, jumping, or coughing as fluid from inflammation irritates the peritoneum. Abdominal pain may or may not be accompanied by fever, nausea, vomiting, diarrhea, anorexia, or dysuria. Often the challenge in diagnosing appendicitis is the variability of clinical presentation. Young children under 5 years of age are particularly difficult to diagnose since they are less able to communicate location and nature of their pain. These children may present only with vague signs of discomfort and, as a result, these patients have higher rates of perforation.

On physical exam, patients commonly present with tenderness to palpation in the RLQ at McBurney's point, which is one-third of the distance between the anterior superior iliac spine and the umbilicus. Several other physical exam maneuvers may be helpful in the evaluation of a child for possible appendicitis. The obturator sign, obtained by internally rotating a flexed hip, will elicit pain when an inflamed appendix comes into contact with the obturator muscle. The psoas sign, performed by extending the right thigh while the patient lies on the left side, will elicit pain when an inflamed appendix overlies the psoas muscle. Rovsing's sign describes pain felt in the RLQ of the abdomen with palpation of the left lower quadrant due to stretching of the peritoneum causing pain in the area of inflammation. Rebound tenderness in the RLQ may also be elicited with deep palpation of the abdomen followed by quick withdrawal of pressure and is also due to right-sided peritoneal irritation. These signs alone are not sufficiently sensitive or specific for diagnosis of appendicitis, but they are helpful when used in conjunction with other signs and symptoms in the evaluation for appendicitis. In a patient with a clear history and physical exam, the diagnosis of appendicitis may be made clinically. However, when there is diagnostic uncertainty and appendicitis remains on the differential diagnosis, further evaluation with laboratory tests and/or imaging is required.

Laboratory tests such as white blood cell (WBC) counts and C-reactive protein (CRP) levels are commonly obtained in children with suspected appendicitis. However, the utility of these tests is limited. The sensitivity and specificity of the WBC count for diagnosis of appendicitis range from 60% to 100% and 20% to 53%, respectively.[2] WBC counts and CRP levels are nonspecific systemic inflammatory markers, and they must be used and interpreted in clinical context for the evaluation of appendicitis. Other laboratory tests that may be obtained in a patient with abdominal pain include hepatic function tests, lipase, urinalysis, and human chorionic gonadotropin in females of reproductive age. Laboratory testing should be limited and done thoughtfully. However, any female of reproductive age must be tested to exclude pregnancy.

Imaging modalities, such as ultrasonography (US), computed tomography (CT), and magnetic resonance imaging (MRI), are helpful when there is diagnostic uncertainty for appendicitis, particularly in pediatric patients that may not present with a typical history or physical examination. In recent years, US has become increasingly utilized as the first-line imaging modality to evaluate RLQ pain due to its lack of ionizing radiation, lower cost, ability to obtain dynamic imaging, elimination of the need for administration of contrast, and no need for sedation. In a recent multicenter study, US was shown to have an overall sensitivity of 73% and specificity of 97% in diagnosis of appendicitis.[3] If the appendix is not visualized directly, secondary signs of inflammation in the RLQ on US may suggest pathology. Emergency department point-of-care ultrasound (POCUS) for appendicitis, performed and interpreted at the bedside by the clinician, has been shown to have similar accuracy as radiology-performed ultrasound, and a positive POCUS may eliminate the need for further imaging while a negative POCUS does not exclude appendicitis.[4] If an US is nondiagnostic and the appendix is not visualized in a patient with concern for appendicitis, CT and MRI have higher accuracy and are more definitive tests for evaluation of appendicitis, with MRI being preferred in pediatrics due to the ionizing radiation associated with CT scans. MRI and CT are very useful tools in the work-up of acute appendicitis and may uncover alternate diagnoses for the etiology of the patient's abdominal pain. However, patients need to be able to stay still to obtain imaging, which may be for a substantial amount of time in the case of MRI, and younger children may require sedation. In a recent study, unenhanced MRI has been shown to have very high diagnostic accuracy when used as first-line diagnostic imaging in children with acute abdominal pain.[5] Alternatively, a surgery consult may be obtained and/or a patient may be observed with serial abdominal examinations to evaluate for progression or resolution of symptoms.

Once a diagnosis of appendicitis is made, antibiotics should be administered expeditiously and a surgical consult should be called. While surgery is currently the definitive treatment for acute appendicitis, studies of children treated nonoperatively suggest that antibiotics may halt the progression of appendicitis to perforation.[6] In addition, a few studies have demonstrated the efficacy and safety of nonoperative treatment for both uncomplicated and complicated appendicitis, with efficacy rates of 71% to 94%.[7] While nonoperative management of appendicitis has gained more traction outside of the United States and in adult populations, there is evidence that antibiotic management of appendicitis may be well tolerated and a reasonable management strategy in select pediatric populations.

In addition, a meta-analysis noted a significant reduction in wound infections and intra-abdominal abscesses among children and adults undergoing appendectomy who received antibiotic prophylaxis.[8] Piperacillin-tazobactam or a combination of metronidazole and ceftriaxone are two common antibiotic regimens used to cover enteric organisms that cause infection in appendicitis. In cases of complicated appendicitis, defined as perforated appendicitis with or without formed abscess or phlegmon, a course of antibiotics is given to treat the infection. Per surgery recommendations, either an appendectomy is done near the time of diagnosis or percutaneous drainage of the abscess is done with the patient returning a few weeks later for an interval appendectomy.

In addition to antibiotic therapy, pain control should also be a mainstay of treatment before and after a diagnosis of appendicitis is made. Pain management should be guided by the patient's assessment of his or her pain severity whenever possible. Intravenous opioids, such as morphine, are typically a good choice and should be considered prior to US imaging as the US exam may cause pain if pressure on the ultrasound probe is needed to displace bowel gas in order to elicit a good image. While opioid analgesics decrease pain in patients with acute surgical pathology, they do not "mask" physical exam findings or delay time to diagnosis and should be administered appropriately to alleviate a patient's pain in a timely manner.[9]

Overall, children with acute appendicitis who are diagnosed and treated appropriately have good outcomes. With appropriate antibiotic administration and advances in surgical technique, children may no longer be rushed to the operating room and instead may go to the operating room in the next available opening or the next day with no increase in rate of complications, often with same day or next day discharge from the hospital. Complications such as perforation are more often seen in younger children who cannot communicate their symptoms or patients that wait more than 48 hours to seek medical care for their symptoms.

In the case of this patient, with the concern for appendicitis based on his history and physical examination, laboratory tests were obtained and he had an intravenous line placed for fluids and pain control. His laboratory tests were significant for a WBC count elevated to 18,000/μL and

CRP elevated to 11 mg/L. The rest of his laboratory tests, including hepatic function tests, lipase, and urinalysis, were within normal limits. He received a dose of morphine for pain prior to his US exam. The US showed an appendix dilated to 9 mm with a fecolith and surrounding inflammation but no evidence of perforation. A surgery consult was called, and metronidazole and ceftriaxone and intravenous fluids were started. In the morning he went to the operating room for a laparoscopic appendectomy for acute appendicitis. He tolerated the procedure well and went home later that evening.

KEY POINTS

- Appendicitis classically presents as acute onset RLQ abdominal pain.
- Variation in presentation can make diagnosis challenging and requires the clinician to consider a broad differential diagnosis.
- Laboratory studies such as complete blood count and CRP have limited utility in the evaluation for appendicitis.
- Imaging is an important tool in the diagnosis of appendicitis, with ultrasound first line for evaluation of RLQ pain in children.
- Pain management should be considered early and does not alter clinical examination or delay time to diagnosis in appendicitis.
- Early diagnosis, administration of antibiotics, and surgical consultation lead to good outcomes for pediatric patients.

Further Reading
1. Schneider C, Kharbanda A, Bachur R. Evaluating appendicitis scoring systems using a prospective pediatric cohort. *Ann Emerg Med.* 2007;49(6). doi:10.1016/ j.annemergmed.2006.12.016
2. Beltran MA, Almonacid J, Vicencio A, et al. Predictive value of white blood cell count and C-reactive protein in children with appendicitis. *J Pediatr Surg.* 2007;42:1208–1214.
3. Mittal MK, Dayan PS, Macias CG, et al. Performance of ultrasound in the diagnosis of appendicitis in children in a multicenter cohort. *Acad Emerg Med.* 2013;20:697–702.
4. Benabbas R, Hanna M, Shah J, Sinert R. Diagnostic accuracy of history, physical examination, laboratory tests, and point-of-care ultrasound for pediatric acute

appendicitis in the emergency department: a systematic review and meta-analysis. *Acad Emerg Med*. 2017;24:523–551.

5. Mushtaq R, Desoky SM, Morello F, et al. First-line diagnostic evaluation with MRI of children suspected of having acute appendicitis. *Radiology*. 2019;291:170–177.

6. Stevenson MD, Dayan PS, Dudley NC, et al. Time from emergency department evaluation to operation and appendiceal perforation. *Pediatrics*. 2017;139:e20160742.

7. López JJ, Deans KJ, Minneci PC. Nonoperative management of appendicitis in children. *Curr Opin Pediatr*. 2017;29:358–362.

8. Andersen BR, Kallehave FL, Andersen HK. Antibiotics versus placebo for prevention of postoperative infection after appendicectomy. *Cochrane Database Syst Rev*. 2005;3:CD001439. doi:10.1002/14651858.CD001439.pub2

9. Aghamohammadi D, Gholipouri C, Hosseinzadeh H, Khajehee MA, Ghabili K, Golzari SE. An evaluation of the effect of morphine on abdominal pain and peritoneal irritation signs in patients with acute surgical abdomen. *J Cardiovasc Thorac Res*. 2012;4(2):45–48.

11 Tummy Ouchie

Nkeiruka Orajiaka and Meghan Dishong

An 18-month-old, previously healthy female presents
to the emergency department with 6 hours of
intermittent episodes of abdominal discomfort. Her
mother describes her as having on and off episodes
of crying and drawing legs up to her abdomen
in discomfort. She is recovering from an upper
respiratory infection which started about 5 days ago.
She has had 2 looser, non-bloody bowel movements
today but no vomiting. She does not have a history of
hard stools or foul-smelling urine.

On examination, patient is afebrile with a
temperature of 99.1°F, heart rate of 120, respiratory
rate of 32, and blood pressure of 88/56 mmHg. She
appears non-toxic but drowsy. Her abdominal exam is
full and soft with no palpable masses and no obvious
discomfort. A few minutes after completing your
exam, you are called to the room with concerns of the
patient having an episode of screaming and she is in
obvious discomfort.

What do you do now?

DISCUSSION

Abdominal pain in a toddler can be challenging, even to the most astute and experienced physician. The differential is usually broad as children this age generally cannot localize pain and parents may have a difficult time knowing where the child is hurting and therefore they present with vague complaints such as fussiness or not acting right. An accurate abdominal exam on patients in this age group can be challenging, as they are well into the stage of stranger anxiety and are likely to start protesting your exam before you even lay a stethoscope on them. Having a well-defined differential facilitates a focused history and physical exam, prior to determination of diagnostic testing. Frequently, abdominal pain in this age group is caused by constipation as they commonly eat diets low in fiber and may have poor water intake. Constipation may be exacerbated during toilet training, by the child withholding stool. Another, less common diagnosis that should be high on the differential for this patient is intussusception. Intussusception classically presents with colicky, episodic abdominal pain with periods in between which the patient either returns to baseline or becomes drowsy. Another critical diagnosis is acute appendicitis. As just discussed, young children often will not localize their abdominal pain so the classic right lower quadrant pain is typically absent. Features that this patient lacks for appendicitis include no fever, no vomiting, and the fact that the symptoms only started 6 hours ago. A urinary tract infection may be easily missed in a toddler and is an important consideration in a female with abdominal pain. Gastroenteritis, viral or bacterial, can cause significant abdominal pain, and in some cases pain occurs first and other associated symptoms such as vomiting and diarrhea occur subsequently.

Creating a differential diagnosis should help you decide and prioritize the child's evaluation in the emergency department. Imaging is a valuable tool in the evaluation of a child with episodes of abdominal pain. Abdominal radiographs are important to evaluate for the possibility of small bowel obstruction or pneumoperitoneum and may also provide a visual image of the stool burden in constipation. Abdominal ultrasound is the gold standard for diagnosis of intussusception and can also be used to diagnose cases of acute appendicitis. A urinalysis may also be considered and would be a reasonable test to perform.

With this patient's history and witnessed paroxysm of pain, intussusception is suspected and an abdominal radiograph and an ultrasound are obtained. The abdominal x-ray is suggestive for intussusception given the lack of bowel gas in the right lower quadrant, and the abdominal ultrasound confirms the diagnosis (Figure 11.1).

Intussusception is one of the most common abdominal emergencies in children, typically occurring between ages 6 to 36 months. It is a process of intestinal obstruction that occurs when one part of the intestine telescopes into a distal portion of the intestine. The part of the intestine that telescopes is usually proximal and is called the intussusceptum, while the receiving distal part is the intussuscipiens. The most common type is ileocolic, but ileo-ileal and colo-colic also can occur.

The typical patient is an infant or toddler presenting with intermittent episodes of colicky abdominal pain during which the child may appear uncomfortable and strain, coil, and draw up his or her knees toward the abdomen. In between episodes the patient may appear normal or may become tired and drowsy. The classic triad for intussusception involves abdominal colic and an abdominal mass and red currant jelly stools (but this only occurs in approximately 1 in every 5 patients with intussusception). Vomiting is another common presenting sign and may occur with

(a) (b)

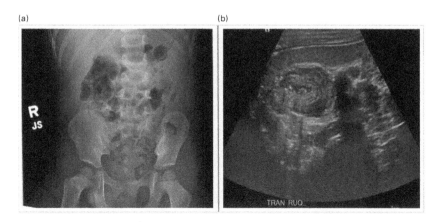

FIGURE 11.1. (a) Abdominal Radiograph: Note the paucity of air in the right lower quadrant (RLQ) and the increased density over the mid to right upper quadrant (RUQ). (b) Ultrasound limited to Intussusception: Note the multiple concentric target sign of the intussusceptum inside an intussuscipiens.

the abdominal pain or occur alone. With progression of the obstruction, pressure increases within the wall of the intussusceptum, causing venous drainage to become impaired and subsequently arterial flow is compromised leading to bowel ischemia. The intestinal mucosa sloughs off and mixes with blood and mucous and appears as black or red currant jelly stool. This is usually a late finding. Abnormal behavior or lethargy may also be the only presenting symptom for intussusception in much younger children, making the diagnosis very challenging. Patients with a prolonged presentation may also come into the emergency department with findings of septicemia and dehydration.

Appropriate history and physical examination can suggest the process of intussusception, but a high index of suspicion is necessary in atypical presentations. The gold standard for diagnosis of intussusception is abdominal ultrasound. This relatively inexpensive and noninvasive tool has a reported sensitivity and specificity of about 100%. In facilities with limited ability to obtain an immediate ultrasound, an abdominal radiograph can be an initial imaging study. A radiograph suggestive of intussusception may show an elongated soft tissue mass, typically in the right upper quadrant, and a paucity of gas showing the collapsed distal intestinal segment, which is typically in the right lower quadrant. Laboratory work up is usually not necessary but may be done in atypical presentations or in severe cases for evaluation of electrolyte imbalances or septicemia.

Intussusception is an abdominal emergency and management should proceed forward as soon as possible. Nonoperative enema reduction is usually the initial preferred method of management with absolute contraindications being intestinal perforation or evidence of peritonitis. Pneumatic and hydrostatic enemas have replaced the barium enemas as the first-line intervention in most institutions. Both pneumatic or air enemas and hydrostatic enemas have been shown to have a higher success rate when compared to barium enemas. Studies have found the success rate for air and hydrostatic enemas to be between 80% and 90%. An air enema involves injecting air into the rectum with interventional radiology to assess for successful reduction. A hydrostatic reduction is another alternative, and various fluids have been used for this procedure including saline, lactated ringer's solution, or tap water. The nonoperative reduction is performed under ultrasound guidance so there is no radiation involved. Either image-guided hydrostatic or pneumatic enema reductions are acceptable options with choice of procedure being institutionally dependent. It is recommended that patients be hydrated using intravenous fluids prior to reduction attempts, or this can be done concurrently so as not to delay time to reduction.

While there is a high success rate for air and hydrostatic enemas, not every case is able to be efficaciously reduced. One study assessed the risk factors for an unsuccessful reduction and found that patients with symptoms lasting greater than or equal to 48 hours; patients who were less than 1 year of age; and patients with constipation, rectal bleeding, or a presence of an abdominal mass on the left side of the abdomen all had an increased risk for failure with hydrostatic reduction. Controversy exists regarding the timing of surgical intervention. Some advocate for surgical intervention after the first failed attempt. Others, however, recommend one or two more attempts under the postulation that first attempts can partially reduce the intussusception, making the intussusceptum less edematous and improving venous drainage, thereby making a second attempt at reduction more successful. One study found that there was a significant increase in the success rate of a delayed reduction attempt if the initial enema provided enough partial reduction such that the leading edge of the intussusception moved to the ileocecal valve. The interval between enemas has not yet been established and may range from 30 minutes to several hours. The rate for successful reduction for each repeat enema varies between 50% and 70%. The risk factors found to increase the risk for an unsuccessful first reduction do not appear to be contraindications for delayed reduction attempts. A maximum number of enema attempts does not appear to have been determined as of yet. A decision must weigh the benefits of avoiding the operating room with the risks of necrotic bowel development if the reduction is delayed. Surgical management is performed in unsuccessful nonoperative reductions and in cases where there are contraindications to nonoperative management.

While the treatment for ileocolic intussusception has been investigated and recommendations are fairly straightforward, the management for ileo-ileal or small bowel-small bowel intussusception can be a bit more controversial. With the increased use of ultrasound, the presence of intussusception in other parts of the bowel is becoming more apparent and the question now is: how benign are these cases? While most cases of ileo-ileal can be managed with observation and supportive care, a small percentage of small bowel intussusceptions require surgical intervention. One recently published study showed that if patients have a history of prior abdominal surgery or focal abdominal pain on exam, then they had an increased risk for a surgical small bowel intussusception (SSBI), but this study also recognized that given the rare occurrence of SSBI, a larger study would be beneficial to corroborate their findings.

Variability also still exists in post-reduction care of children with intussusception. Feeding and monitoring times after nonoperative management differ between institutions. Some patients are advanced to feeds as tolerated while others are placed in fasting to rest the bowel and prevent recurrence. Several studies have suggested no significant benefit to withholding feeds in conscious and stable patients post-reduction, and there is no added risk of recurrence or other complications from early feeding. Recent recommendations have been to commence feeds as tolerated in a conscious patient within 2 hours post-reduction of intussusception.

CONCLUSION

With the patient's confirmed ultrasound diagnosis of intussusception, she was placed on a nil per oral status; intravenous hydration commenced with normal saline, and the pediatric surgery team was consulted. Air enema reduction was successfully done after 2 attempts under diagnostic ultrasound. Both reduction attempts were within a period of 1 hour and the patient was stable throughout the diagnostic reduction. She was observed in the emergency department for 2 hours post-procedure and was able to tolerate oral fluids with no vomiting or abdominal pain symptoms. She was discharged home and had no return visits for any complications or repeat intussusception.

KEY POINTS

- Abdominal pain in a toddler can be a challenging chief complaint and one should always consider intussusception in the differential.
- The classic triad of symptoms only occurs in 1 out of 5 patients with intussusception.

- Ultrasound is the method of choice for diagnosis of intussusception but a plain radiograph can be helpful.
- Treatment for intussusception involves enema reduction with either air or fluids under ultrasound guidance or fluoroscopy.

Further Reading

1. West KW, Stephens B, Vane DW, Grosfeld JL. Intussusception: current management in infants and children. *Surgery*. 1987;102:704–710.
2. Beasley SW. The "ins" and "outs" of intussusception: where best practice reduces the need of surgery. *Journal of Paediatrics and Child Health*. 2017;53:1118–1122.
3. Pazo A, Hill J, Losek JD. Delayed repeat enema in the management of intussusception. *Pediatric Emergency Care*. 2010;26:640–645.
4. Xiaolong X, Yang W, Qi W, Yiyang Z, Bo X. Risk factors for failure of hydrostatic reduction of intussusception in pediatric patients: a retrospective study. *Medicine*. 2019;98:1–6.
5. Sandler AD, Ein SH, Connolly B, Daneman A, Filler RM. Unsuccessful air-enema reduction of intussusception: is a second attempt worthwhile? *Pediatric Surgery International*. 1999;15:214–216.
6. Vandewalle RJ, et al. Radiographic and clinical factors in pediatric patients with surgical small-bowel intussusception. *Journal of Surgical Research*. 2019;233:167–172.
7. Adekunle-Ojo AO, Craig AM, Ma L, Caviness AC. Intussusception: postreduction fasting is not necessary to prevent complications and recurrences in the emergency department observation unit. *Pediatric Emergency Care*. 2011;27:897–899.
8. Forati S, Yaghmaii B, Allah-Verdi B. The effect of early feeding after enema reduction of intussusception in order to investigate the rate of recurrence and side effects of reduction. *Biomedical Research*. 2017;28:13.
9. Melvin JE, et al. Management and outcome of pediatric patients with transient small bowel-small bowel intussusception. *Pediatric Emergency Care*. 2018. Advance online publication.

12 Another Day, Another GI Bug

Pinaki Mukherji and Dana Libov

A 9-month-old, full-term, previously healthy, vaccinated male presents with recurrent abdominal pain and vomiting over the last 2 months. A consultation with the pediatrician 1 month ago resulted in a recommendation to begin H2 blocker treatment for possible reflux. One week prior, the child vomited, but the child resumed feeding normally within 2 days. Now the parent states that the child appears unwell, is unable to tolerate any oral intake, and has vomited 6 times in the past 24 hours, with 1 episode of slightly loose stool. Vital signs reveal an afebrile child with HR 130, BP 70/40, RR 32, POx 100% RA. Your exam reveals an otherwise well-developed child who has dry mucous membranes, is slightly irritable with both parent and provider, and has a soft abdomen with mild distention, normal bowel sounds, and no rebound or guarding but grimaces to any palpation of the abdomen.

What do you do now?

DISCUSSION

The presentation of gastrointestinal complaints in children is both commonplace and overall remarkably benign. Many will be correctly diagnosed as having viral syndromes or simple dietary intolerance. Only patients who are failing expectant management and are becoming significantly symptomatic will undergo aggressive testing and evaluation. This child requires hydration (whether oral or parenteral), basic laboratory testing, and repeat abdominal exams.

SCENARIO 1

Oral hydration attempts fail, and an intravenous cannula is placed with an initial 20 mL/kg fluid bolus order. A glucose point of care test is performed, which is your common practice in caring for ill pediatric patients, and is reported at 35. You order a 5 mL/kg infusion of D10W. The child is less irritable but not tolerating oral liquids even after anti-emetics. Repeat abdominal exam is improved. Review of labs further reveals an aspartate aminotransferase (AST) of 122, an alanine aminotransferase (ALT) of 38, and metabolic acidosis with an anion gap.

WHAT DO YOU DO NOW?

This child is a likely admission at this point for continued symptomatic treatment, with maintenance fluids, repeat glucose testing, and serial anion gap measurements. The combination of metabolic acidosis and hypoglycemia suggests sepsis but also stirs a recollection of that category of diseases referred to as inborn error of metabolism (IEM) and an ammonia, lactate, and uric acid is added to the laboratory testing. The elevated ammonia level strengthens the suspicion of an IEM.

Diagnosing IEM is a challenging prospect, with subtle presenting symptoms and time of onset varying greatly among this group of diseases which now number more than 40 distinct entities. IEM encompasses disorders including organic acidurias, urea cycle defects, fatty acid oxidation defects, and glycogen storage disorders, to name a few. For the emergency provider, appreciating the presenting symptoms and ordering initial screening will allow more rapid diagnosis by subspecialists. IEM can present in a variety of different ways including poor feeding, vomiting, respiratory complaints (tachypnea or apneic periods), and generalized weakness or lethargy. Testing may reveal hypoglycemia, hyperammonemia, liver dysfunction, myopathy, or acidosis. The constellation of findings can be used to guide the work-up, utilizing different algorithms depending on varying symptoms at presentation and lab findings (see Figure 12.1).

After IEM is suspected and the work-up is under way, management is disease specific but treatment should not be withheld until a definitive diagnosis is possible. Broadly, presumptive management should include reducing toxic metabolites, liberal glucose administration to prevent catabolism and utilization of metabolic pathways, and targeted cofactor administration based on the category of IEM suspected. While a specific diagnosis may not be immediately available, a broad category based on a constellation of screening lab abnormalities is quite possible.

While many patients with IEM present in the newborn or neonatal period, delayed diagnoses can occur. This patient presented at 9 months of age, later than most IEM, but has a typical history concerning for aminoacidopathy, with worsening episodic vomiting. Symptoms may begin later in life and can occur up to 1 year of age with this IEM due to the advancing of diet and introduction of new proteins. The combination of metabolic acidosis and hyperammonemia triggered suspicion for IEM testing which ultimately diagnosed the patient with the rare condition HMG-CoA lyase deficiency. The child was placed on a restricted leucine diet and began carnitine therapy, with dialysis held in reserve for potential worsening hyperammonemia and encephalopathy.

KEY POINTS

· Think of inborn errors of metabolism in newborns and during the first month of life, but some presentations can be delayed.
· Screen for IEM by testing glucose, ammonia, lactate, ketones, and uric acid.

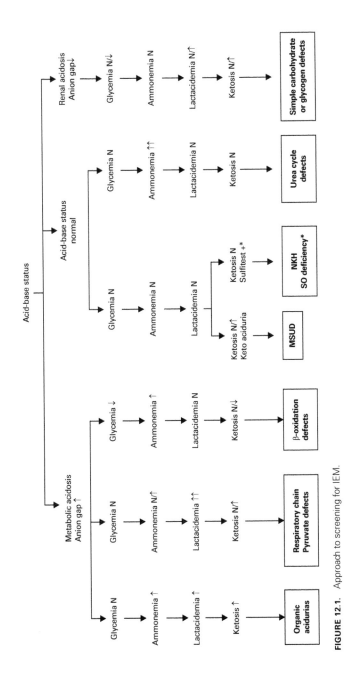

FIGURE 12.1. Approach to screening for IEM.

- Sepsis is a common misdiagnosis- the younger the child, the more you should consider IEM.
- Reye's syndrome is a common misdiagnosis—some Reye's patients have been diagnosed with underlying fatty acid oxidation disorders. (Reye's syndrome incidence is falling so IEM is currently statistically more likely).

SCENARIO 2

As oral rehydration is initiated, the patient vomits a small amount of liquid; however, using a 10 ml syringe allows for a 10 mL/kg fluid challenge in the first hour. The abdominal exam continues to show diffuse mild tenderness and the patient continues to be irritable when examined. The patient's lab testing shows an AST of 122, an ALT of 38, and a lipase of 190. The parent is asking whether he will be ready for discharge soon, since "last time after he drank, we were fine at home."

WHAT DO YOU DO NOW?

The persistently tender exam and abnormal labs raise concern for an underlying medical issue, so the decision is made to reassess the child's vital signs. The nurse repeats vital signs at the bedside and asks you to look at a small ecchymosis at the child's left flank above the anterior superior iliac spine. The combination of the lab findings and the bruise triggers you to think of nonaccidental trauma (NAT). A skeletal survey is performed showing healed left-sided 7th and 8th posterior rib fractures.

NAT continues to account for mortality in 2/100,000 children, and 74% of cases involve children less than 3 years of age. Child Protective Services data indicates that neglect accounts for most referrals, but physical and sexual abuse represent nearly 30% of cases, with head trauma most highly associated with mortality. Any injury to a non-ambulatory child should have NAT as part of the differential diagnosis, and unfortunately the presentation may be very subtle, especially in younger, nonverbal children. Features in the history that should raise suspicion of NAT, including changing HPIs, delayed presentations, and mechanism of injury not matching objective injury patterns.

The skin is a commonly injured organ, and bruises are not "minor" injuries. Bruising to the head or trunk or over any non-bony areas is suspicious even in older children, while any bruising anywhere in nonambulatory patients should raise concern. Clustering of bruises to certain areas and regular patterns or shapes are highly suspicious. The timing of an injury cannot be determined from the appearance of the ecchymosis, but multiple bruises of different appearance and color may be an indicator of NAT. Historical concerns or skin injuries that are concerning should prompt a skeletal survey. Fractures, the second most common injury in NAT, are categorized from high to low suspicion, with sternal, scapular, spinous process, and rib fractures carrying the highest specificity for NAT. The "bucket-handle" metaphyseal fracture is commonly seen in NAT as well, occurring in the proximal humerus, distal femur, and proximal or distal tibia. Spiral fractures are suspicious in nonambulatory children for NAT but are not considered highly suspicious in older children with a history consistent with injury.

Although abdominal injury secondary to NAT has been previously reported as rare, recent epidemiologic data from hospitalized children in the United States shows that NAT accounts for more than one-fourth of all hospitalizations for abdominal trauma in children younger than 1 year of age. In infants and children aged 0 to 4 years, abuse accounts for at least 15% of blunt abdominal injuries. Additionally, abdominal injury in NAT is frequently severe with higher rates of exploratory laparotomy and a six-fold increase in the odds of death. If there is suspicion for abdominal trauma, urinalysis and computed tomography (CT) scanning with contrast is recommended. Lab findings associated with blunt trauma include abnormal liver function tests and lipase; however, these are not sensitive enough to be used as screening tests. Brain imaging should be considered in patients with head injury or abnormal neurologic exams as well, either CT or magnetic resonance imaging (MRI) of the brain. Since abusive head trauma accounts for ~80% of mortality in NAT, there is a low threshold to investigate if injury is uncertain. CT is generally more readily available and can be performed quickly. Utilizing MRI may increase delays to imaging and cost, but it is a more sensitive test that can be useful prognostically in head trauma and diagnostically when a diagnosis of diffuse axonal injury is being considered.

A report is placed to Child Protective Services, as is required by law in all U.S. states, and it is explained to the parent that the child will be admitted because of his injuries. In addition to the skeletal survey ordered, CT imaging of the abdomen is also obtained. The younger age and irritability of the patient prompts an order for a CT of the brain as well. While the presumptive diagnosis in this case is NAT, after discussion with the inpatient team a parallel medical workup is ordered which includes a coagulation panel, platelets, calcium, phosphorus, alkaline phosphatase, parathyroid hormone, d-dimer, fibrinogen, and factor VIII and IX levels. The pediatric team will follow these to assess for bleeding disorders and bone health.

KEY POINTS

- Most injuries in children are not due to neglect or NAT, but up to 10% of the emergency department populace of pediatric trauma may be related to NAT.
- Preverbal patients are at highest risk for NAT with the greatest mortality in children 0 to 3 years of age.
- Bruises to non-bony areas, especially ears, abdomen, upper arms, or thighs, are red flags. Oral, dental, or genital injuries are also suspicious.
- Lipase, AST, and glucose have been shown to be elevated in blunt trauma with an elevated lipase carrying the highest positive predictive value.
- When initiating screening, consider adding lab diagnostics and advanced imaging including CT or MRI to the skeletal survey.
- Emergency providers are mandated reporters of suspected NAT to Child Protective Services or a state authority.

SCENARIO 3

When attempting oral and parenteral rehydration, the patient now has an episode of witnessed bilious vomiting. The patient receives lab testing showing an AST of 122, ALT of 38, chloride of 92, potassium of 2.8, and

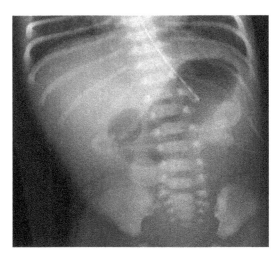

FIGURE 12.2. Two discrete areas of distention, paucity of bowel gas elsewhere. "Double bubble sign."

Young, JR. Feb 2015 Creative Commons licensed, Wikimedia commons.

pH of 7.46. Repeat abdominal exam is unchanged though patient appears progressively more irritable, prompting an abdominal x-ray. An abdominal radiograph demonstrates dilated stomach and small bowel (Figure 12.2). An ultrasound is ordered, which is nonspecific but comments on dilated loops of bowel.

WHAT DO YOU DO NOW?

The bilious vomiting and abdominal radiograph (double bubble sign), in concert with hypochloremia and hypokalemic metabolic alkalosis are the most concerning features of this case. Potential diagnosis include necrotizing enterocolitis (presents early in infancy, bloody stool, pneumatosis intestinalis) and pyloric stenosis (non-bilious emesis, olive on palpation, hypokalemic, hypochloremic metabolic alkalosis). A careful examination of the genitalia will exclude an incarcerated hernia and torsion. The combination of the radiograph (double bubble sign) with the laboratory studies strongly suggests malrotation with volvulus. Surgical consultation and management focused on stabilization should be pursued. Fortunately, this patient remains hemodynamically stable and advanced imaging can be obtained for definitive diagnosis.

Malrotation is a congenital anatomic anomaly that has a 2:1 male predominance. While many with malrotation are symptomatic within the neonatal period, only 58% of patients present by 1 year of age. Malrotation occurs because of failure of appropriate rotation of midgut around the superior mesenteric artery during embryonic development. This leads to a narrow base of mesentery which promotes an environment for the mesentery to twist around the SMA, leading to volvulus. The presentation is typically acute but can be subacute in nature, with recurrent episodes of vomiting suggestive of intermittent volvulus consistent with this patient's previous episodes of poor feeds. Midgut volvulus can present insidiously and similarly to many other serious diagnoses, so prompt diagnosis is needed. Persistent volvulus is a surgical emergency, however, because it will lead to bowel ischemia and necrosis.

Upper gastrointestinal series is the gold standard in pediatric patients for volvulus, but if the diagnosis is suspected, treatment should not be delayed. The abdominal radiograph performed suggests a "double bubble" sign, which is very suggestive of midgut volvulus. Ultrasound and CT can also aid in the diagnosis, but lack sensitivity, and considerations such as radiation exposure should be considered given alternate diagnostic options.

In a patient with possible malrotation and midgut volvulus, a nasogastric tube should be placed, antibiotics administered, and an emergent call to the pediatric surgeon on call placed. If CT imaging is obtained, the radiologist may indicate that a "whirl" or "whirlpool" sign is present, showing a twisting of the mesentery around the superior mesenteric artery (Figure 12.3), which has been described on ultrasound imaging as well. Patients undergo a Ladd's procedure—a detorsion maneuver and surgical division of Ladd's bands widening the mesentery, treating the obstruction and preventing recurrent volvulus.

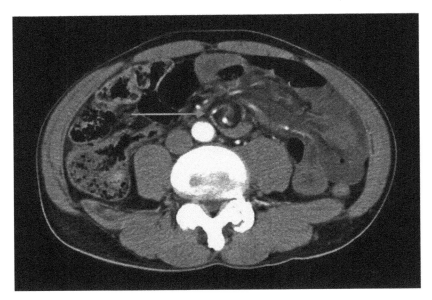

FIGURE 12.3. "Whirl" or "whirlpool" sign.
Takeshi K, Kazuhiko T. Midgut volvulus. *BMJ* 2017 Mar;356:i6782.
Reproduced with permission from BMJ.

KEY POINTS

- Bilious vomiting is suggestive of obstruction and can represent malrotation with midgut volvulus in the pediatric population.
- A "whirlpool" sign on CT imaging is suggestive of midgut volvulus.
- Examine an infant's genitalia to make sure a torsion or incarcerated hernia are not missed.
- Focus in the emergency department is acute stabilization and emergent surgical consultation with a pediatric surgeon.
- Delays in diagnosis can lead to bowel necrosis and increase morbidity and mortality.

Further Reading

Applegate KE. Evidence-based diagnosis of malrotation and volvulus. *Pediatr Radiol.* 2009;39(S2):S161–S163.

Burton BK. Inborn errors of metabolism in infancy: a guide to diagnosis. *Pediatrics.* Dec 1998;102(6):e65.

Capraro AJ, Mooney D, Waltzman ML. The use of routine laboratory studies as screening tools in pediatric abdominal trauma. *Pediatric Emerg Care*. 2006 Jul 22(7):480–484.

Christian CW. The evaluation of suspected child physical abuse. *Pediatrics*. 2015 May;135(5):e1337–e1354.

Kimura K., Loening-Baucke V. Bilious vomiting in the newborn: rapid diagnosis of intestinal obstruction. *Am Fam Physician*. 2000;61(9):2791–2798.

Mak CM, Lee HC, Chan AY, Lam CW. Inborn errors of metabolism and expanded newborn screening: review and update. *Crit Rev Clin Lab Sci*. 2013 Nov. 50(6):142–162.

Nehra, D., Goldstein AK. Intestinal malrotation: varied clinical presentation from infancy through adulthood. *Surgery*. 2011;149:386–393.

Paul AR, Matthew AA. Non-accidental trauma in pediatric patients: a review of epidemiology, pathophysiology, diagnosis, and treatment. *Transl Pediatr*. 2014 Jul 3(3):195–207.

Sizemore, AW., Rabbani, KZ., Ladd, A. et al. Diagnostic performance of the upper gastrointestinal series in the evaluation of children with clinically suspected malrotation. *Pediatr Radiology*. 2008;38:518.

Weiner DL. Inborn errors of metabolism. In Aghababian RV, ed. *Emergency medicine: the core curriculum*. Philadelphia: Lippincott-Raven; 1999.

13 What's This Pounding in My Head?

Sakina Sojar and Lauren Allister

A 12-year-old female presents to the emergency department with headaches that started 4 months ago and have been progressively worsening in severity and increasing in frequency over the last 2 months. The headaches are throbbing in character, and she occasionally has photopsia and nausea. Over the last week, she has also had intermittent vision loss. She has been using ibuprofen daily for her symptoms with minimal relief. Her past medical history is notable for acne. Her mother and older sister have a history of migraine headaches.

On physical exam she is alert and oriented. Her fundoscopic exam is notable for bilateral papilledema and a 6th nerve palsy in her right eye. Her visual acuity testing is normal, but she does experience intermittent diplopia on exam. Her sensation is grossly intact. Her strength is 5/5 throughout. Her gait is normal. The remainder of her exam is unremarkable.

What do you do now?

DISCUSSION

Headaches in the pediatric population are a common presentation in primary care offices and emergency departments. Headache etiologies are divided into two categories: primary headaches, which are due to an intrinsic condition (e.g., migraines, tension headaches, chronic headache, and cluster headaches) and secondary headaches, which are due to an acquired condition (e.g., sinus congestion, abnormal intracranial pressures, idiopathic intracranial hypertension, infection, vascular malformation, and space-occupying lesions). Headaches most commonly present in postmenarchal adolescent females, but they can be seen in patients of any age. Though the majority of pediatric headaches are non-life-threatening, they are associated with significant morbidity, including truancy, stress, and parental anxiety. The provider is often faced with the challenge of delineating whether the headache requires a work-up with laboratory studies and/or neuroimaging. In most cases pediatric headaches can be managed symptomatically with pharmacotherapy and lifestyle changes.

Neuroimaging and further studies should be acquired in the presence of "red flag" signs and symptoms (Table 13.1). On history these include early morning headaches, persistent early morning vomiting, worsening headaches, new onset headaches within the last 6 months, headaches that wake a patient from sleep, altered mental status, or seizures. On physical exam these include any focal neurological deficits, a Glasgow Coma Score less than 15, or an abnormal fundoscopic examination. Fever, neck stiffness, persistent vomiting,

TABLE 13.1. **Red Flag Symptoms Warranting Consideration of Imaging**

History	Physical Exam
Early morning headaches	Focal neurological deficits
Early morning vomiting	GCS <15
Worsening headaches	Abnormal fundoscopic examination
New onset in <6 months	Papilledema
Wake from sleep	Cushing's Triad
New onset seizure	Altered mental status

Note. GCS = Glasgow Coma Scale.

and sepsis should prompt concern for meningitis or encephalitis requiring acquisition of cerebrospinal fluid and initiation of empiric broad-spectrum antibiotics. The combination of hypertension, bradycardia, and an irregular breathing pattern is known as Cushing's triad and suggests increased intracranial pressure and impending brainstem herniation. In our patient's history, the presence of progressively worsening headaches, recent headache onset in the last 4 months, and vision loss as well as the exam findings of papilledema and a cranial nerve deficit warrants neuroimaging.

Computed tomography (CT) and magnetic resonance imaging (MRI) are the two primary imaging modalities used to evaluate for neurological disease. CT scans of the brain have several advantages. Images can be obtained within minutes, they are relatively inexpensive, and patients often will not require sedation for image acquisition. Unfortunately CT scans expose patients to significant radiation, which may have deleterious long-term effects. Conversely an MRI provides a high-resolution image with zero radiation exposure. However, an MRI is time-intensive and cost-prohibitive and can sometimes detect incidental findings that may not be clinically relevant. Other considerations in choosing the appropriate neuroimaging modality include contraindications to contrast dye or gadolinium.

CT scan is an optimal choice when neuroimaging is needed rapidly, when evaluating headaches secondary to trauma, when there is a need to assess ventricle size, or when there is concern for an acute, life-threatening vascular lesion. This patient who presents with a new focal neurological deficit (sixth nerve palsy) would warrant an initial emergent non-contrast CT of the head to rule out one of these life threatening diseases. CT angiography may also be valuable in these scenarios. MRI can obtain better resolution of the brain parenchyma and will better evaluate for malignancies, masses, venous thromboses, lesions, autoimmune disease, and meningeal inflammation. Rapid sequence MRI protocols (not requiring sedation) have been developed at many institutions primarily to evaluate for hydrocephalus in patients with concern for ventricular shunt malfunction or infection. On average, these rapid protocols take 3 minutes to obtain and can provide valuable information such as ventricle size, ventricle configuration, and presence of the shunt catheter. The reduced exposure to ionizing radiation from repeated CT scans as well as reduced exposure to sedation is extremely valuable in this population that require repeated imaging of the brain. Further research is addressing whether rapid MRI sequences may be of value for other indications to assess for hydrocephalus or other intracranial pathologies in healthy children.

The history and exam in this case are consistent with intracranial idiopathic hypertension (IIH), formerly known as pseudotumor cerebri. IIH occurs when there is increased intracranial pressure in the absence of ventriculomegaly or other sequelae of another secondary neurological disease. IIH is most common in obese, postpubertal females, though can also occur in younger, non-obese children. It presents with progressively worsening headaches, transient visual symptoms, photopsia, back pain, neck pain, and pulsatile tinnitus. Medications used to treat acne, specifically tetracyclines and tretinoin, are known to put patients at risk for this condition. Visual symptoms are caused by the compression of the optic nerve and can be permanent if IIH is not recognized and treated. Physical exam will be significant for papilledema (Figure 13.1), with or without cranial nerve III, IV, or VI palsies. A fundoscopic exam is critical in helping to differentiate the need for imaging, though sometimes a difficult skill to obtain in young patients. Any additional neurological deficits on exam should prompt consideration of an alternative diagnosis. IIH should be considered a diagnosis of exclusion, as the differential for intracranial hypertension is broad and contains many life-threatening diagnoses. The ultimate imaging modality of choice for IIH is MRI.

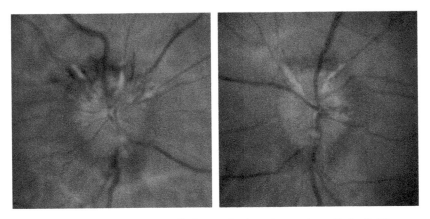

FIGURE 13.1. Presence of bilateral papilledema on fundoscopic exam in a patient with IIH.

It is important to note that another headache type on the differential diagnosis for this patient is migraine headache. Migraine headaches typically have a pulsatile character of pain, which is generally moderate to severe in intensity. Nausea, vomiting, photophobia, and phonophobia frequently accompany them. A family history of migraines is often present. Acute first-line treatment for migraine headache includes abortive therapy with a nonsteroidal anti-inflammatory drug (NSAID) or a triptan, an antiemetic, and fluids. Second-line therapies, such as magnesium, caffeine, valproate or steroids may be indicated in certain cases. Chronic NSAID use, as exhibited in the case, can paradoxically worsen the frequency and severity of migraine headaches. Long-term management of migraine headaches comprises of lifestyle modification +/− maintenance pharmacotherapy. Lifestyle modifications include normalization of sleep patterns, elimination of caffeine or caffeine withdrawal, and avoidance of skipping meals. In the emergency department setting, patients are generally treated with intravenous (IV) ketorolac, IV prochlorperazine, and IV fluids. Patients with complex migraines can have concomitant auras, vertigo, paralysis, and inability to focus or decreased cognitive functioning, prompting a physician to consider the need for neuroimaging. Acute neuroimaging is not routinely required in evaluating patients with migraine headaches.

When IIH is suspected, the work-up should begin with an MRI of the brain to rule out any secondary causes of increased intracranial pressure. For most patients with this disease, the MRI of the brain will be normal. Ventricle size should not be enlarged. Neuroimaging may reveal an empty sella, enhancement of the optic nerve, or flattening of the posterior sclera.

After secondary causes of headaches have been excluded by neuroimaging, the definitive diagnostic and therapeutic step for IIH is a lumbar puncture with measurement of opening pressure. The opening pressure must be obtained in the lateral decubitus position with the legs extended. A value higher than 26 cmH$_2$0 (normal opening pressure is 18 cmH$_2$0 to 20 cmH$_2$0) is diagnostic of the disease. Cerebrospinal fluid (CSF) should be sent for cell count, protein, and glucose. At the time of measurement, CSF should be removed therapeutically as a means to relieve pressure on the optic nerve. Medical management includes the initiation of a carbonic anhydrase inhibitor, most commonly acetazolamide. Acetazolamide decreases the production of cerebrospinal fluid at the choroid plexus. Weight loss in obese patients may also help provide symptomatic relief.

Patients who have persistent symptoms despite these measures are at risk for permanent vision loss. Surgical options to be considered are optic nerve sheath fenestration or ventricular shunt placement. Prognosis in IIH varies among patients. Monthly ophthalmologic exams are recommended at the onset of diagnoses to follow progression of disease and prevent permanent vision loss.

KEY POINTS

- The majority of pediatric headaches do not require imaging. Imaging should be considered when red flag symptoms are noted on history or physical exam.
- Imaging modalities to choose from include CT scan of the head or MRI of the brain. CT scans allow for rapid image acquisition but expose patients to radiation. MRI of the brain allows for high resolution and superior images, however, may require the use of sedation and the test itself is time consuming to obtain and perform in most hospital settings.
- Rapid MRI protocols are a novel method of evaluating for ventriculomegaly or mass effect and may eliminate the need for sedation and exposure to radiation.

Further Reading

1. Alexiou G, Argyropoulou M. Neuroimaging in childhood headache: a systematic review. *Pediatr Radiol.* 2013;43(7):777–784. doi:10.1007/s00247-013-2692-3
2. Blume H. Pediatric headache: a review. *Pediatr Rev.* 2012;33(12):562–576. doi:10.1542/pir.33-12-562
3. Kelly M, Strelzik J, Langdon R, DiSabella M. Pediatric headache. *Curr Opin Pediatr.* 2018;30(6):748–754. doi:10.1097/mop.0000000000000688
4. Kirkham F. Indications for the performance of neuroimaging in children. *Handb Clin Neurol.* 2016;136:1275–1290. doi:10.1016/b978-0-444-53486-6.00065-x
5. Schobitz E, Qureshi F, Lewis D. Pediatric headaches in the emergency department. *Curr Pain Headache Rep.* 2006;10(5):391–396. doi:10.1007/s11916-006-0066-3

6. Thurtell M, Tomsak R, Daroff R. *Neuro-ophthalmology*. New York, NY: Oxford University Press; 2011. doi:10.1093/med/9780195390841.001.0001

7. Mercille G, Ospina L. Pediatric idiopathic intracranial hypertension. *Pediatr Rev*. 2007;28(11):e77–e86. doi:10.1542/pir.28-11-e77

8. Patel D, Tubbs R, Pate G, Johnston J, Blount J. Fast-sequence MRI studies for surveillance imaging in pediatric hydrocephalus. *J Neurosurg Pediatr*. 2014;13:355–470. doi:10.3171/2014.1.peds13447

9. Charles A. Migraine. *N Engl J Med*. 2017;377(6):553–561. doi:10.1056/nejmcp1605502

14 Why Is My Child Shaking All Over?

Katherine Battisti

A previously healthy 3-year-old female arrives to the emergency department by ambulance along with her frightened parents. The parents report that the patient was sitting in her mother's lap reading a book before bed when her arms and legs started shaking and her eyes rolled back. This lasted for approximately 10 minutes during which the child did not respond to the parents' attempts to get her attention. They called for emergency services who arrived shortly before the shaking stopped without intervention, after which time the patient was sleepy and confused. The patient slowly improved over the next 45 minutes and now on exam has returned to her neurologic baseline and has normal vital signs.

What do you do now?

DISCUSSION

The approach to a seizing patient begins with determining if the patient is still seizing, with an initial focus on airway, breathing, and circulation. Patients who are seizing or postictal often have airway compromise and may require airway repositioning such as a jaw thrust or neck roll. Bag mask ventilation and intubation can also become necessary, particularly if the seizure is difficult to control. Associated apnea either due to the seizure or to the anti-epileptic medications patients have received can occur. Circulation is more likely to be compromised after anti-epileptic drugs have been administered as several of the medications result in decreased vascular tone and potentially hypotension.

While managing the stabilization of the patient, attempt to get the seizures under control if they are persistent. Start abortive medications if seizures last longer than 5 minutes to prevent progression to status epilepticus. The ultimate goal is to prevent complications including brain injury, hyperthermia, rhabdomyolysis due to muscle breakdown, and death. Nearly universally, providers agree that first-line abortive medications are benzodiazepines, typically midazolam (0.05–0.1 mg/kg intravenous [IV] max 10 mg or 0.2 mg/kg intranasal [IN] max 10 mg) or lorazepam (0.05–0.1 mg/kg IV max 4 mg). For infants in the first few months of life, the second-line treatment is phenobarbital (20–40 mg/kg IV loading dose). In older patients, second-line treatment is often fosphenytoin (20 mg/kg IV), which is better tolerated than phenytoin; however, randomized control studies are currently underway to compare the efficacy of (fos)phenytoin, levetiracetam, and valproic acid. In the event of treatment failure after multiple medications, patients often require continuous IV drips of benzodiazepines or phenobarbital. Early consultation with neurology or intensive care colleagues is indicated if management requires the use of multiple medications as these patients often need intubation and admission.

In addition to managing ongoing seizures, consider if additional work-up is indicated keeping in mind the differential (Table 14.1). The history and physical exam of the seizing patient is incredibly important in determining the next steps of the evaluation and management. What laboratory testing or neuroimaging is needed for a patient with a history of developmental delay is different than the work-up for a febrile patient or a patient

TABLE 14.1. **Differential Diagnosis for New Onset Seizures in Pediatric Patients**

Hypoxic Ischemic Encephalopathy[†]

Hemorrhagic Stroke

Ischemic Stroke

Intracranial Hemorrhage

  Intraventricular Hemorrhage

  Parenchymal Hemorrhage

  Subarachnoid Hemorrhage

  Subdural Hemorrhage

Hydrocephalus

Congenital Brain Malformation[†]

Infection

  Meningitis

  Encephalitis

  Brain Abscess

  Congenital (TORCH*) Infection[†]

  Sepsis

Malignancy

Nonmalignant Space Occupying Lesions

  Ex. Tubers from Tuberous Sclerosis

Autoimmune Disorder

Trauma

Metabolic Derangement

  Hypoglycemia or Hyperglycemia

  Hypocalcemia

  Hyponatremia[†]

Benign Febrile Seizures

TABLE 14.1. **Continued**

Epileptic Disorders

Inborn Errors of Metabolism[†]

  Hyperammonemia

  Hyperglycemia

Kernicterus[†]

Vascular Malformations

Increased Intracranial Pressure

Hypertension

Toxic Exposure

Idiopathic

---

* TORCH = Toxoplasmosis, Other (syphilis, parvovirus B19), Rubella, Cytomegalovirus, Herpes Viruses.
† Typically presents within the first 6 months of life.

who has a history of epilepsy. Age also plays an important role in the differential for the underlying etiology of a first-time seizure. Neonates up to a corrected age of 44 weeks gestation with seizures have been found to have significant pathology in 76% of cases including genetic disorders, inborn errors of metabolism, infection, ischemic or hemorrhagic stroke, or congenital malformations. Hypoglycemia and hypocalcemia account for another 10% of cases. Infants less than 12 months of age with a first-time seizure remain more likely to have underlying genetic or metabolic conditions, congenital brain abnormalities, or pre-existing brain insult than children who present at an older age. Similarly, the physical exam can help direct the evaluation and management. A patient who returns to neurologic baseline after a brief postictal period requires less evaluation than one who remains in status epilepticus or who is somnolent for a prolonged period of time. Focal neurologic findings after the post ictal period also warrant more extensive evaluation. Other physical exam findings such as numerous café au lait spots, ash leaf spots, or a facial port wine stain may indicate a higher likelihood of intracranial abnormalities that require further investigation as well.

One of the easiest ways to approach the evaluation of a patient with a seizure is to divide patients into different categories of seizures. These categories include the following: simple and complex febrile seizures, first non-febrile seizure, known epilepsy, and status epilepticus.

Simple and complex febrile seizures can usually be treated the same way although more thought should be given to the evaluation of a patient with a complex febrile seizure. Simple febrile seizures are seen in up to 5% of pediatric patients and are defined as a single generalized seizure lasting less than 15 minutes in a patient between the ages of 6 months and 5 years of age accompanied by a temperature of 100.4°F (38°C) or higher within a 24-hour period. In contrast, complex febrile seizures are febrile seizures in patients between the ages of 6 months and 5 years that are either focal, last longer than 15 minutes, and/or are recurrent within a 24-hour period. The fever needs to be within 24-hours of the seizure, but it does not need to occur simultaneously and not uncommonly the fever develops hours after the seizure. If the patient returns to his or her neurologic baseline, little to no work-up is indicated for the seizure regardless if the febrile seizure is simple or complex.

The job of the emergency provider is to evaluate the patient with febrile seizures for the underlying infection as indicated by the history and exam and to treat the infection accordingly. If the exam is suggestive of meningitis or encephalitis (e.g., nuchal rigidity, a bulging anterior fontanelle, toxic appearance, or persistent altered mental status), a lumbar puncture is indicated. If the patient is under-vaccinated (particularly for *Hemophilus influenzae type b* or *Streptococcus pneumonia*), or the patient has been pretreated with antibiotics, a lumbar puncture should be considered. No laboratory testing or imaging is indicated unless diagnostically needed to identify an underlying infection (urinalysis, chest x-ray, or influenza testing). Neuroimaging is not indicated unless there are signs or symptoms suggestive of brain abscess, increased intracranial pressure, or hemorrhage. While the literature remains controversial, neuroimaging prior to lumbar puncture for patients in whom increased intracranial pressure is suspected is advised in the setting of patients with seizures. Notably, neuroimaging is often obtained in patients with focal seizures, status epilepticus, or a prolonged postictal period; however, the utility is very low. It is also important to note that febrile patients who do not fit into the 6 months to 5 years age range are excluded from this recommendation, so higher suspicion for intracranial infection is warranted and lumbar puncture should be more strongly considered. Additionally, if the patient has a history of afebrile seizures, the work-up should be tailored to evaluation of the underlying infection as fevers are known to increase the likelihood of seizures in patients with underlying epilepsy even when they are otherwise well controlled.

First-time unprovoked, non-febrile seizures in pediatric patients, in contrast with adult patients, often require no emergent laboratory evaluation or neuroimaging. Pediatric patients often undergo extensive evaluation in the emergency department due to provider discomfort. This is costly and largely unnecessary in most cases. Evaluation of these patients should be tailored to their history. Neuroimaging is indicated in patients who have a focal neurologic deficit after their seizure that does not resolve rapidly and in patients who do not return to baseline. There is a significantly higher incidence of abnormal neuroimaging in patients less than 2 years of age. A history of prematurity, birth complication, or unexplained developmental delay is also associated with increased likelihood of abnormal neuroimaging. The decision between an emergent computed tomography or a prompt outpatient magnetic resonance imaging (MRI) should be based on the stability of the patient, recurrence of seizure activity, focality of the seizure, or status epilepticus. Unlike with febrile seizures, laboratory evaluation can be useful in patients with afebrile seizures particularly focusing on hypoglycemia, hyponatremia, and hypocalcemia. Electrolyte abnormalities are of the highest yield in infants less than 1 year of age as well as in children in status epilepticus. In children with a possible intentional or accidental ingestion, toxicology screening may be indicated as well. An electroencephalogram (EEG) should be done, but in a stable patient with return to neurologic baseline this can be done nonemergently as an outpatient. Infants less than 6 months of age with recurrent seizures warrant admission for observation and further evaluation even if they return to baseline between seizures, due to the higher rate of abnormalities on either laboratory evaluation or neuroimaging in these patients.

In patients with known epilepsy, unless there is evidence of a new neurologic change, neuroimaging is typically not indicated emergently. Exceptions to this would include patients with intracranial shunts in place. A lower threshold for imaging should also be considered in patients with known intracranial malignancy or patients with high risk of stroke such as patients with sickle cell disease, systemic lupus erythematosus, or Moyamoya disease. Laboratory testing should be limited to medication levels of anti-epileptic drugs for the purposes of determining compliance and if the patient is within therapeutic levels.

The patient in the vignette is a previously healthy 3-year-old who returns to baseline after a brief postictal period. This is consistent with a first-time afebrile seizure; however, keep in mind that this could be a febrile seizure if fever develops within the next 24 hours. After a period of observation during which the patient's history is reviewed and a return to neurologic baseline is confirmed, this patient can be discharged home with no emergent laboratory or imaging evaluation. Education on seizure safety, especially the avoidance of unsupervised swimming/bathing or putting objects in the patient's mouth, should be provided to the family prior to discharge. If the patient remains afebrile, she will need an outpatient neurology evaluation, likely including an EEG and possibly an MRI at the discretion of a neurologist. Arranging a follow-up with the child's pediatrician within 24 hours of the emergency department evaluation may facilitate outpatient referrals and a repeat evaluation.

Knowing what the indications are for evaluation of patients with seizures that fall into the different categories can reduce the cost of evaluations, risk of unnecessary radiation exposure, and unnecessary transfer and admissions for most patients. A summary of the recommendations can be found in Table 14.2.

TABLE 14.2. **Summary of Recommendations by Seizure Category**

Seizure Category	Recommended Approach to Evaluation
Simple and Complex Febrile Seizures	• Obtain laboratory testing/imaging only as indicated for the evaluation of underlying infection • Obtain lumbar puncture only if exam suggestive of meningitis/encephalitis • Obtain neuroimaging only if signs/symptoms of brain abscess, increased intracranial pressure or hemorrhage • EEG is not indicated
First Nonfebrile Seizure (Unprovoked)	• Obtain laboratory testing if indicated by history/physical, including electrolytes and toxicology screening • Obtain lumbar puncture only if exam suggestive of meningitis/encephalitis • Neuroimaging indicated for patients with signs of increased intracranial pressure, hemorrhage, neurologic deficits, and delayed return to baseline. In stable patients imaging can be done outpatient. Highest yield in patients less than 2 years of age • EEG indicated but can be done outpatient
Known Epilepsy	• Laboratory testing only to check medication levels unless specific concern for electrolyte disturbance • Neuroimaging not indicated unless patient with ventricular shunt or new neurologic abnormalities

KEY POINTS

• Patients who return to their neurologic baseline often require no laboratory or neuroimaging evaluation in the emergency department.
• Children less than 6 months of age with seizures should be admitted for observation and further evaluation under the guidance of a neurologist.
• Febrile seizures occur in patients between 6 months and 5 years of age. Patients with a classic febrile seizure require only a

diagnostic evaluation for an underlying infection as guided by the history and physical exam.

- The indication for laboratory evaluation including lumbar puncture is based on history and physical exam, particularly the physical exam after postictal period.
- Neuroimaging should be pursued in patients with persistent focal neurologic deficits, signs of increased intracranial pressure, persistent altered mental status, status epilepticus, or suspicion of trauma.
- Neuroimaging should be considered in patients with new focal seizures and children less than 2 years of age.

Further Reading

Al-shami R, Khair AM, Elseid M, et al. Neuro-imaging evaluation after the first afebrile seizure in children: a retrospective observational study. *Seizure*. 2016;43:26–31.

Aprahamian N, Harper MB, Prabhu SP, et al. Pediatric first time non-febrile seizure with focal manifestations: Is emergent imaging indicated? *Seizure*. 2014;23:740–745.

Hsieh DT, Chang T, Tsuchida TN, et al. New-onset afebrile seizures in infants: role of neuroimaging. *Neurology*. 2010;74:150–156.

Lawton B, Deuble N. Seizures in the paediatric emergency department. *J Paediatr Child Health*. 2016;52:147–150.

Ronen GM, Penney S, Andrews W. The epidemiology of clinical neonatal seizures in Newfoundland: a population-based study. *J Pediatr*. 1999;134(1):71–75.

Santillanes G, Luc Q. Emergency department management of seizures in pediatric patients. *Pediatr Emerg Med Pract*. 2015;12(3):1–25.

Subcommittee on Febrile Seizures, American Academy of Pediatrics. Clinical Practice Guideline—Febrile seizures: guideline for the neurodiagnostic evaluation of the child with a simple febrile seizure. *Pediatrics*. 2011;127(2):389–394.

15 Shaking for More than Five

Nina Ackerman

A 5-year-old boy with no significant past medical history presents with a tonic-clonic seizure. History is obtained from the mother and emergency medical services (EMS). The patient had been well up until 2 days ago, when he developed fever, cough, sore throat, and runny nose. He has been receiving acetaminophen and ibuprofen as needed. Today the patient was home playing in the living room, when suddenly he started rhythmically jerking his arms and legs. The mother called EMS, who arrived and administered 2 mg intramuscular (IM) midazolam. When the child arrives at the emergency department, he appears lethargic and minimally responsive. Vital signs are HR 128 bpm, RR 20 breaths/min, BP 105/70, O2 sat 96%, Temp 39.4°C, and fingerstick glucose is 92. Physical exam reveals a lethargic child who otherwise appears healthy. There are no signs of trauma and no rashes. He has clear lungs and a soft, and nontender abdomen. After the exam is completed the patient starts to seize again.

What do you do now?

DISCUSSION

Seizures, or hyperactivity of a group of cortical neurons causing a behavioral change in a patient, are a common neurologic disturbance in children and can be triggered by a wide variety of causes. The incidence of status epilepticus in children vary by age, with the highest incidence in the neonatal period and then declining until approximately 5 years of age. A higher incidence occurs in vulnerable populations with acute or chronic neurologic conditions.

The 2015 International League Against Epilepsy defines status epilepticus as

> a condition resulting either from the failure of the mechanisms responsible for seizure termination or from the initiation of mechanisms which lead to abnormally prolonged seizures. It is a condition that can have long-term consequences (after time point t_2), including neuronal death, neuronal injury, and alteration of neuronal networks, depending on the type and duration of seizures.

Time points were variably defined based on whether the seizure was generalized tonic-clonic status epilepticus, focal status epilepticus with impaired consciousness, or absence status epilepticus. Their definition recognizes the variable urgency in treating status epilepticus based on the type of seizure, distinguishing between status epilepticus with motor features and without prominent motor features. The 2012 Neurocritical Care Society's Guideline on the Evaluation and Management of Status Epilepticus defines status epilepticus as 5 minutes of continuous clinical or electrographic seizure activity. The 2016 American Epilepsy Society's Guideline for Status Epilepticus Management follows the 5-minute definition without subdividing based on seizure type. Prolonged or recurrent seizures have a high morbidity and mortality, therefore, seizures lasting 5 or more minutes require emergent intervention. Aborting seizures can decrease neurologic sequelae and the frequency of future episodes of status epilepticus as well as improve clinical outcomes. The length of the seizure and the refractoriness of response to treatment will usually correspond to morbidity and mortality. Neurologic sequelae of seizures can include focal neurologic deficits, paralysis, cognitive impairment, developmental delays, and behavioral disturbances. A careful history is very important and can aid in treatment. Other diagnoses to consider that can easily be mistaken for seizures are syncope, breath-holding spells, migraine with aura, movement disorders, and behavioral disturbances. A postictal period, or persistent altered mental status, tongue-biting, and incontinence, are signs that point the diagnosis toward seizure.

Once the diagnosis of seizure is made, the top priorities in a child who has persistent seizure activity are managing the airway and aborting the seizure. The child in the case study presents with recurrent tonic-clonic activity. The first priority will be assessing and stabilizing the patient's airway and positioning the child to maximize oxygenation and ventilation and prevent aspiration, usually on his side. Apply nasal cannula or non-rebreather and suction secretions as necessary. If there are obvious signs of airway compromise, the seizing child should be intubated. Intravenous (IV) access and vital signs should be obtained quickly so that any abnormality can be addressed. Continuous cardiac monitor and pulse oximetry should be instituted.

Rapidly correctable etiologies for status epilepticus benefit from early identification and emergent treatment and include hypoglycemia, hypocalcemia, hyponatremia, and hypomagnesemia. The American Academy of Neurology practice parameter reported abnormal results among children who underwent testing including low anti-seizure medication levels (32%), neuroimaging abnormalities (8%), electrolytes (6%), inborn errors of metabolism (4%), ingestion (4%), central nervous system infections (3%), and positive blood cultures (3%) (Riviello et al., 2006). To identify precipitants, the Neurocritical Care Society's guideline recommends a finger-stick glucose in the initial 2 minutes. In addition, recommended testing includes a serum glucose, complete blood count (CBC), comprehensive metabolic panel (CMP), blood gas, calcium, magnesium, and anti-seizure medication levels drawn in the first 5 minutes (Brophy et al., 2012).

For hypoglycemia a bolus of D10 at 5 mL/kg should be given and rectal acetaminophen as well as cooling blankets can be administered for fever. The child in the scenario has a glucose of 92, so no glucose is given.

Once the ABCs are addressed, anticonvulsant treatment should be initiated and the patient should be reassessed for seizures every 5 minutes (see Figure 15.1). First-line anticonvulsants are benzodiazepines, lorazepam,

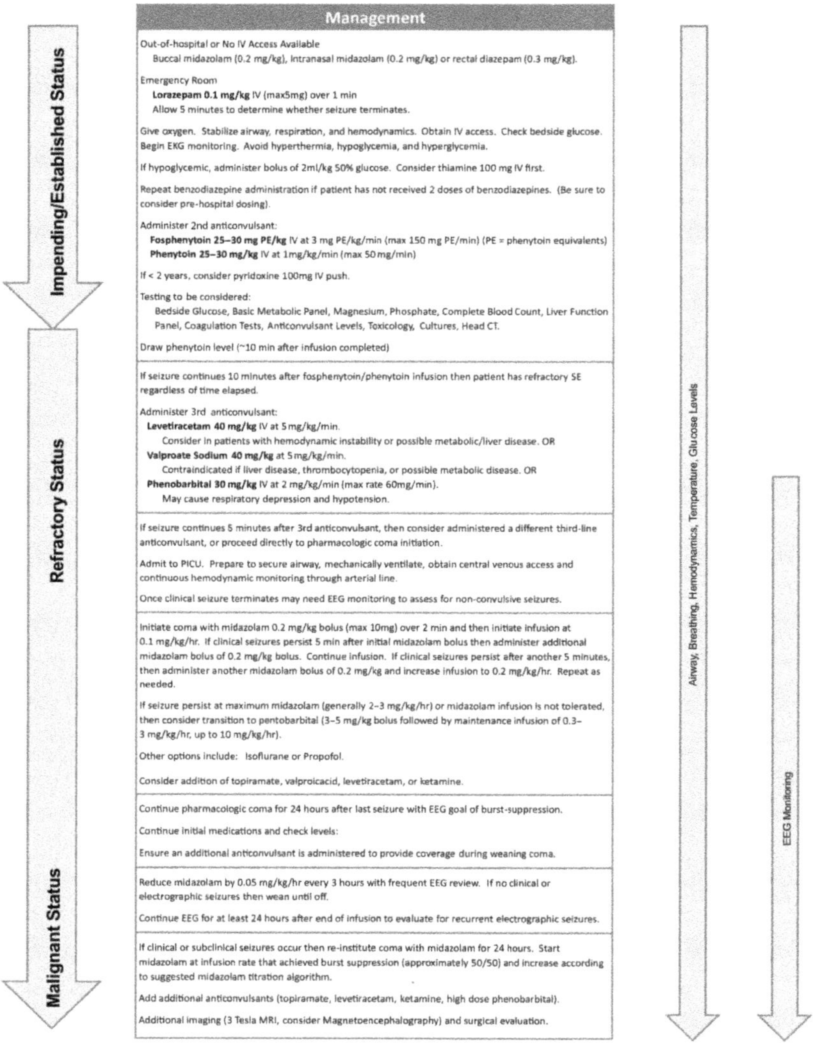

FIGURE 15.1. Management of status epilepticus in children. Figure from Abend NS, Guitierrez-Colina AM, Dlugos DJ. Medical treatment of pediatric status epilepticus. *Seminars in Pediatric Neurology*. 2010;17:169. Used with permission.

diazepam, or midazolam. If IV/intraosseous infusion access is not obtained, midazolam 0.1–0.2 mg/kg IM, 0.2 mg/kg buccal, or intranasal 0.2 mg/kg can be used. If seizures continue after 5 minutes, a second dose of benzodiazepines should be given. The child in the scenario is given a second dose of midazolam, but the seizure activity persists.

After 2 doses of benzodiazepines are administered without aborting seizure, urgent control antiepileptic drug (AED) therapy recommendations include use of IV fosphenytoin/phenytoin, valproate sodium, or levetiracetam. The patient should be loaded with fosphenytoin 20 mg phenytoin equivalents (PE)/kg at a rate of 3 PE/kg/minute. The Neurocritical Care Society's guideline classifies phenytoin and fosphenytoin as appropriate emergent, urgent, or refractory status epilepticus treatments.

Valproic acid is effective in the treatment of both generalized and focal epilepsy and may be more effective in treating status epilepticus in children than in adults (Trinka, 2007). In two recent meta-analyses, valproic acid was found to have the highest relative efficacy among typical second-line anti-seizure medications. Valproate may be administered rapidly intravenously and is classified as an appropriate "emergent," "urgent," or "refractory" status epilepticus medication by the Neurocritical Care Society's guideline.

Phenobarbital may be used as indicated by the Neurocritical Care Society's guideline as an "emergent," "urgent," or "refractory" status epilepticus medication. The typical intravenous loading dose is 20 mg/kg, with an additional 5–10 mg/kg if needed. A recent meta-analysis of drugs administered for benzodiazepine refractory convulsive status epilepticus found that phenobarbital was efficacious in 74% of patients. Phenobarbital is sedating and may result in respiratory depression or hypotension.

Levetiracetam is an additional antiseizure medication option to be considered for urgent therapy. Recent data suggests it may be useful for early status epilepticus due to its ease of dosing and lack of drug interactions. A meta-analysis of drugs administered for benzodiazepine refractory convulsive status epilepticus found levetiracetam was efficacious in 69% of subjects.

If there is suspicion that the patient may be taking isoniazid, pyridoxine can be administered as well for isoniazid poisoning. Phenobarbital can cause apnea and respiratory depression, especially in conjunction with multiple doses of benzodiazepines, so the child most likely will require airway support, including intubation.

If the patient persists with seizure activity, the Neurocritical Care Society's guideline indicates one of two options: administering a bolus of an unused urgent control medication and then proceeding to pharmacologic coma induction if seizures persist, or moving directly to pharmacologic coma induction. Additional urgent control antiseizure medications (e.g., phenytoin, valproate, levetiracetam, and phenobarbital) are reasonable considerations if seizures are decreasing in frequency. Very little data is available regarding management of refractory status epilepticus with midazolam, pentobarbital, or other anesthetic therapies. Propofol may rapidly terminate seizures, but it is rarely used in children due to its Federal Drug Administration black box warning due to propofol infusion syndrome.

More recently, studies are suggesting that a ketamine bolus of 2–3 mg/kg followed by a continuous infusion at 7.5 mcg/kg/h can be used as a third line for refractory status epilepticus. Ketamine has fewer side effects than phenobarbital and does not cause respiratory depression, possibly avoiding the need for endotracheal intubation. There are ongoing studies to further elucidate the benefit and efficacy of ketamine as an antiepileptic.

Once the seizure is controlled and the patient is stabilized, further assessment and physical exam should be completed and a thorough history should be taken. The most common causes of seizures in children include fever, infections, medications, toxic ingestion, metabolic derangements, tumor, intracerebral hemorrhage or infarct, neurocutaneous disorders, and epilepsy, among others.

Signs or symptoms of infection or illness preceding the seizure can clue the provider about etiology of the seizure and guide further work-up. Febrile seizures are the most common cause of status epilepticus and typically occur in children ages 6 months to 6 years. Febrile seizures, in contrast to fever-induced seizures, are in children who do not have a history of seizures without fever. Fever can lower the seizure threshold in a child who has an underlying seizure disorder and provoke a seizure. The most common viruses associated with febrile seizures are HHV-6, HHV-7, and influenza. Central nervous system infections, like meningitis or encephalitis, need to be considered as a cause of seizure as well and may be hard to differentiate from a febrile seizure. In many cases, especially if the child has not returned to his baseline mental status, lumbar puncture is indicated to rule out a more severe infection and antibiotics should be administered.

A history of recent trauma, or nonaccidental trauma, should be considered particularly in younger, nonverbal children. Any suspicion for trauma warrants further workup with computed tomography (CT) scan. Any medications the patient has access to, including his own or family members, should be reviewed, as toxic ingestions or withdrawal from medications including antidepressants, anticholinergics, sympathomimetics, anticonvulsants, antipsychotics, and many other agents can cause seizures. Certain antibiotics and other drugs, even when ingested at therapeutic levels, can lower the seizure threshold in a patient with a seizure history as well. In children with a history of seizures, it is important to ascertain level of compliance of AEDs and if there were any missed doses precipitating the seizure.

If possible, send labs, including, complete blood count, comprehensive metabolic test, magnesium, Ph, toxicology screen, and AED levels. Labs are useful in determining if there is a metabolic derangement that can be addressed. In children, inborn errors of metabolism, dehydration, and inappropriate infant formula usage can cause electrolyte disturbances that are associated with seizures, such as hypoglycemia (<40 mg/dL), hyponatremia (<125 mEq/L), and hypernatremia (>150 mEq/L). Hypocalcemia and hypomagnesemia can also cause seizures. Any lab abnormalities should be corrected. In every female of childbearing age, a urine HCG or serum quantitative HCG should be sent. Eclampsia should be considered in a pregnant or postpartum patient with elevated blood pressures and needs to be treated with IV magnesium and urgent obstetrician consultation.

If no clear etiology is ascertained on review of history, physical exam and labs, the patient will likely require neuroimaging (CT/magnetic resonance imaging) to rule out any structural abnormality or a tumor. In many cases this will be normal as well, and status epilepticus may be the first presentation of the epilepsy. In patients who do not have a prior history of epilepsy, EEG is the preferred test and can best elucidate seizure type. Continuous monitoring should ideally be initiated once it is determined that the child is in refractory status epilepticus.

Once the child is stabilized and seizures are aborted, he or she can be dispositioned as appropriate.

In this case, the child receives IV fosphenytoin/phenytoin and the seizure activity terminates. The child receives neuroimaging (which is normal), CBC (normal), and CMP (normal) and is admitted to the hospital. After a 24-hour admission he is discharged home with scheduled follow-up with a neurologist.

KEY POINTS

- Remember to always check blood glucose level first and quickly address hypoglycemia.
- First-line treatment for status epilepticus is a benzodiazepine. Urgent AEDs include fosphenytoin, levetiracetam, valproic acid, or phenobarbital.
- Consider giving pyridoxine for refractory seizures.

Further Reading

Abend NS, Gutierrez-Colina AM, Dlugos DJ. Medical treatment of pediatric status epilepticus. *Seminars in Pediatric Neurology*. 2010 Sep 1;17(3):169–175.

Brophy GM, Bell R, Claassen J, et al. Guidelines for the evaluation and management of status epilepticus. *Neurocritical Care*. 2012;17:3–23.

Gurcharran K, Grinspan ZM. The burden of pediatric status epilepticus: epidemiology, morbidity, and mortality. *Seizure*. 2018;68:3–8.

Marx JA, Hockberger RS, Walls RM. *Rosens Emergency Medicine: Concepts and Clinical Practice* (2 vols.). Philadelphia: Elsevier Saunders; 2014.

Riviello JJ, Ashwal S, Hirtz D, et al. Practice parameter: diagnostic assessment of the child with status epilepticus (an evidence-based review). *Neurology*. 2006;67:1542–1550.

Trinka E. The use of valproate and new antiepileptic drugs in status epilepticus. *Epilepsia*. 2007;48(S8):49–51.

Vasquez A, Farias-Moeller R, Tatum W. Pediatric refractory and super refractory status epilepticus. *Seizure—European Journal of Epilepsy*. 2018;68:62–71.

Vasquez A, Gaínza-Lein M, Fernández IS, et al. Hospital emergency treatment of convulsive status epilepticus: comparison of pathways from ten pediatric research centers. *Pediatric Neurology*. 2018;86:33–41.

16 Sugar and Spice . . . Not Always Nice

Crista Cerrone and Michael J. Stoner

An 8-year-old male with a history of mild intermittent asthma presents to the emergency department (ED) with "fast breathing." Parents report that it started the night prior and they tried his Albuterol MDI, but he did not get much relief from it. He has had rhinorrhea, congestion, and cough over the last 5 days but no fever. The patient reports he started to have stomach pain this morning. The mom has been giving him "lots of fluids to help him pass this illness" and "he's been peeing a ton with all the juice and sports drinks we've been giving." They deny vomiting or diarrhea.

On exam, the patient is tachycardic to 125 bpm, tachypneic to 28 breaths per minute, with 100% oxygen saturation on room air. He is ill appearing but not toxic, a HEENT exam is normal, his lungs are clear to auscultation with good aeration, his heart rate is a little fast but no murmur is noted, and he has good perfusion. His abdominal exam demonstrates generalized abdominal pain on palpation.

What do you do now?

DIAGNOSIS

There are many different disease processes that can cause tachypnea in pediatric patients. Sometimes it is easy to be sidetracked by a patient's past medical history and assume, as in this patient, it is an asthma exacerbation. Trust your clinical skills. Do you hear wheezing? Is he having a hard time moving air, or is the respiratory rate just too fast? Of course you may not hear wheezing in patients with an asthma exacerbation if they have very poor aeration. Make sure you are hearing good air movement on exam before ruling out asthma as a possible diagnosis with the absence of a wheeze. If you are unsure if you are hearing good air movement, consider trialing a dose of albuterol, with or without ipratropium, to see if there is any change in clinical exam. Again, it is very common to only hear wheezing on your repeat exam if your bronchodilator helped improve the patient's aeration, allowing him or her to move enough air to have a wheeze.

In our patient, the bronchodilator did not affect the lung exam. The patient had good air exchange without any crackles on exam and the patient is afebrile, making pneumonia unlikely. Upper airway diseases may also cause tachypnea and respiratory distress. Especially in unimmunized children, a diagnosis you cannot miss is epiglottitis. Unfortunately, epiglottitis can affect children and adults alike, caused by any number of pathogens including H. Influenzae type B, Staph aureus, and Strep pneumonia.[1,2] These patients are typically very ill appearing. Children will typically sit in a tripod position with neck hyperextended and chin pushed forward to reduce airway resistance.[3] They may report a sore throat and progress rapidly to dysphagia, drooling, and severe respiratory distress. High fevers and a muffled "hot potato" voice are common. The patient in this scenario has none of these symptoms and a normal HEENT exam. Providers should take caution not to upset infants and children and should immediately discuss with ENT and anesthesia in order to have a secured airway placed in the operating room due to the significant amount of inflammation making these a particularly difficult airway to establish. Another upper airway obstruction to consider in our 8-year-old patient with tachypnea and respiratory distress is a peritonsillar abscess. These patients will often present with fevers, muffled "hot potato" voice, sore throat, and trismus. On exam, these patients will often have fullness or bulging around the affected tonsil and may have a uvula that is deviated from midline to the opposite side. The patient's normal HEENT exam excludes this diagnosis. Croup is less common in an 8-year-old, as it is usually seen in younger patients. Without any inspiratory stridor, it is unlikely that our patient has croup.

Other factors not to miss are a history of trauma or ingestion/aspiration. Nonaccidental trauma is a very real consideration. Chest wall trauma can cause splinting, tachypnea, and respiratory distress, in a younger nonverbal child, and may be your only presenting symptoms. Foreign body aspiration can be associated with biphasic stridor, wheezing, cough, decreased aeration, and respiratory distress. Chemical or medication ingestions can present with many distinct findings, including tachypnea, cough, and respiratory distress. Without any significant history of trauma or exposure to any medications or household products, trauma, ingestion, and intoxication are not as high on your differential.

Laboratory Studies

At this point, you now have your bedside venous blood gas and chemistries available to you. The venous blood gas comes back at pH 7.15, pCO_2 25, pO_2 64, HCO_2 8. The patient is acidotic, with a pH of 7.15. It appears to be a metabolic acidosis since the bicarbonate is only 8. The CO_2 of 25 shows evidence of some respiratory compensation, thus explaining the tachypnea. While awaiting the Chem 7 results, consider the possible etiologies for a metabolic acidosis.

A helpful schema to think through cases of a metabolic acidosis in terms of pathogenesis is: (a) Is this caused by an increase in acid either generated internally (e.g., lactic acidosis or ketoacidosis) or from an exogenous source such as a toxin (e.g., salicylates or ethylene glycol)? (b) Is this caused by a decreased alkaline (bicarbonate) in the body (e.g., increased gastrointestinal losses or renal tubular acidosis (RTA)? (c) Is this caused by a reduced excretion of acid in the urine (e.g., RTA or renal failure)? Based on the history obtained so far, there is nothing to suggest increased gastrointestinal losses as the family has denied diarrhea. Ingestion is possible but unlikely given the subacute timeline of symptoms. The patient has been urinating a lot, according to the mom, making renal failure unlikely. Symptoms of RTA can be subtle, so it would be hard to exclude without lab work.

The Chem 7 is now available and shows a Na 134, K 4.0, Cl 98, and HCO$_3$ 8. This child has an anion gap (anion gap = sodium – [chloride + bicarbonate], so for this patient 134 – [98 + 8] = 28). High anion gap metabolic acidosis triggers the MUDPILES mnemonic (methanol, uremia, diabetic ketoacidosis, paraldehyde, iron and isoniazid, lactic acidosis, ethylene glycol, and salicylates). The remainder of the Chem 7 includes a BUN 38, Cr 1.0, and glucose 782. So the patient has a hyperglycemic, high anion gap metabolic acidosis, consistent with diabetic ketoacidosis (DKA).

DISCUSSION

About thirty percent of new onset type I diabetes mellitus will present in DKA.[4] DKA is defined as (a) blood glucose > 200 mg/dL; (b) metabolic acidosis: pH <7.30 or bicarbonate <15 mmol/L; and (c) ketosis: beta-hydroxybutyrate >3 mmol/L or "moderate" to "large" urine ketones.[5] It can be distinguished from a hyperglycemic hyperosmolar state because of the acidosis and presence of ketones. Classic presenting features of a patient in DKA are tachycardia, tachypnea, dehydration, deep sighing respirations (Kussmaul respirations), nausea, vomiting, abdominal pain, confusion, drowsiness, and decreased level of consciousness.[5]

MANAGEMENT

Management should always start with evaluation of airway, breathing, and circulation, as with all patients in the emergency department. If a patient is severely obtunded and unable to protect the airway, consider intubating. This is a critical decision as mental status (Glasgow Coma Scale [GCS]) needs to be monitored very closely, and this ability is lost when the child is intubated. This difficult decision is often dependent on resources, ability to monitor, and ability to escalate care. For example, if the patient is to be transported between facilities, a definitive airway should be maintained if at all concerned, whereas a patient in a pediatric intensive care unit might have more latitude as care can be escalated very quickly. It is also important to realize that patients in DKA need to hyperventilate to help prevent even more severe acidosis. If a child in DKA is intubated, he or she must be ventilated at a rate sufficient to allow for respiratory compensation of his or her metabolic acidosis, so try to match the respiratory rate prior to intubation. Although we would typically give a pediatric patient 1 breath every 3 to 5 seconds, for patients with DKA we may give breaths every 1 to 2 seconds to mimic the patient's compensatory breathing.

Once a patient is stabilized, the International Society for Pediatric and Adolescent Diabetes recommends pediatric patients in DKA be treated at a pediatric facility experienced in DKA management.[5] Early involvement of a pediatric hospital may help prevent delays in transfer and allow earlier involvement of pediatric endocrinologists.

MONITORING

The child should be monitored closely with continuous cardiopulmonary monitors and oxygen saturation. He should have a weight obtained to help calculate fluid needs. Even if the patient has recently lost weight, make all fluid calculations based of the patient's current weight. Frequent neurological assessments with GCS scores should be obtained hourly. Patients should be kept NPO with 2 large bore peripheral intravenous (IV) lines placed. Central lines should be avoided as patients with DKA have a high risk of thrombus.[5] If there is a delay in obtaining potassium measurements or if the potassium is high (K >6), providers should consider obtaining an EKG looking for cardiac effects of hyperkalemia.[5]

INITIAL FLUIDS

An initial normal saline bolus (NSB) of 10 to 20 mL/kg should be administered to the patient over 30 to 60 minutes. This presumes patients in DKA are ~5% to 10% dehydrated secondary to increased output (due to glycosuria and increased osmotic diuresis) and decreased intake.[6] An additional 10 mL/kg NSB can be administered thereafter if the patient continues to show signs and symptoms of dehydration. If the patient is in shock, treat with adequate fluids to correct hemodynamic instability.

Insulin

Insulin therapy should begin at least 1 hour after the patient receives the normal saline bolus(es).[5] Insulin should be given via IV infusion at a dose of 0.05 to 0.1 units/kg/hr. Insulin boluses should *never* be administered for DKA in children. Continue the insulin infusion until resolution of DKA (as indicated by pH >7.30, bicarbonate >15, or closure of anion gap).

Fluids While on Insulin

Upon starting an insulin infusion, providers should start fluids with added sodium and potassium based on the initial serum potassium recorded. Glucose will need to be added once the sugar begins to decrease. A two-bag system for the fluids is recommended. One bag will have dextrose (D10) added to the appropriate electrolyte fluids; the other will be without any dextrose. You should start with 100% of the non-dextrose containing fluid, and as the glucose drops below 250 to 300 mg/dL, switch to a 1:1 ratio between the two bags, thus giving you D5, to prevent the glucose from falling into a dangerous range while awaiting the resolution of the DKA. Once the blood glucose falls below 200 mg/dl, switch to using only the D10 bag until the DKA has resolved. During treatment of DKA, aim to have the serum glucose decrease by no more than 100 mg/dL/hour. If the glucose drops quicker than this, you may consider switching to a 1:1 ratio of the two-bag system before the glucose falls below the 250 to 300 mg/dL point. It is important to note that the fluids and insulin are necessary to correct DKA. Thus, if blood sugar decreases too rapidly, it is more appropriate to increase the glucose in the fluids and not decrease the rate of insulin infusion. Decreasing insulin should only be done when the DKA has resolved, or the patient is unable to maintain his blood sugar with maximum glucose in the IV fluids. The initial serum potassium will determine the potassium concentration of the bags (Table 16.1).

The two-bag system should be run at 1.5 to 2 times the patient's maintenance rate. The maintenance rate can be calculated by the 4:2:1 method: (4 ml/kg for the first 10 kg of patient's weight) + (2 ml/kg for the next 10 kg of the patient's weight) + (1 ml/kg for each additional kg of the patient's weight).

Generally, total fluid replacement should be done with a sodium concentration of either 0.9% or 0.45% and should be completed over the subsequent 24 to 48 hours.

TABLE 16.1.   **Recommended Intravenous Fluid Two-Bag System**

If K < 4.5

   Bag 1   0.9% Sodium Chloride or 0.45% Sodium Chloride + 30 mEq/L Potassium Chloride + 30 mEq/L Potassium Phosphate

   Bag 2   D10 0.9% Sodium Chloride or D10 0.45% Sodium Chloride + 30 mEq/L Potassium Chloride + 30 mEq/L Potassium Phosphate

If K = 4.5–6

   Bag 1   0.9% Sodium Chloride or 0.45% Sodium Chloride + 20 mEq/L Potassium Chloride + 20 mEq/L Potassium Phosphate

   Bag 2   D10 0.9% Sodium Chloride or D10 0.45% Sodium Chloride + 20 mEq/L Potassium Chloride + 20 mEq/L Potassium Phosphate

If K > 6

   Bag 1   0.9% Sodium Chloride or 0.45% Sodium Chloride

   Bag 2   D10 0.9% Sodium Chloride or D10 0.45% Sodium Chloride

Note. Intravenous fluid infusion should only be given after the patient has received an initial bolus of normal saline.
D10 = 10% Dextrose.

SERIAL LABORATORY STUDIES

An initial blood glucose should be obtained as well as hourly blood glucoses thereafter. An initial set of serum electrolytes and a blood gas should be obtained, as well as every 2 hours thereafter. When assessing electrolytes, make sure magnesium, phosphate, and calcium are measured at the onset and then every 2 to 4 hours. A rapid rise in serum sodium might indicate the patient is in diabetes insipidus secondary to cerebral injury.[5] A urinalysis to assess for ketones or a serum beta-hydroxybutyrate should be obtained to confirm the diagnosis of DKA. All patients should have a complete blood count. An elevated white blood cell count for these patients is common due to the stress response and does not necessarily indicate an infection. For febrile patients, consider an infection as the body stressor that initiated the episode of DKA. Obtain blood and urine cultures and start appropriate antibiotics if warranted.

COMPLICATIONS

The most common causes of morbidity and mortality in patients with DKA are cerebral edema, arrhythmias secondary to electrolyte disturbances, thrombus, necrotic bowel, renal failure, and Acute Respiratory Distress Syndrome (ARDS).[5] Cerebral edema should be suspected in patients who are obtunded, restless, irritable, or confused. Other signs include worsening or new onset headache while undergoing treatment, cranial nerve palsies, vomiting, or exhibiting Cushing's triad (bradycardia, hypertension, and respiratory abnormalities).[5] Cerebral edema usually occurs within the first 12–24 hours of presentation, but may be present at any time in the course. Treatment of cerebral edema should be done quickly with hyperosmotic therapy. This includes either Mannitol 0.5 to 1 g/kg IV over 10 to 15 minutes or hypertonic saline (3%) 2.5 to 5 mL/kg over 10 to 15 minutes.[7,8] The head of the bed should also be elevated to 30 degrees and providers should consider intubation to maintain the patient's airway if they suspect pending neurologic compromise. Patients should be examined closely and reassessed regularly during the treatment of DKA to recognize and treat the associated complications.

CASE RESOLUTION

This child was diagnosed with DKA. He received a 20 ml/kg fluid bolus in the emergency department, and the two-bag system and insulin therapy were initiated. His glucose was lowered at 100mg/dL per hour. He was admitted and the family was educated on managing his diabetes. He was discharged to home under the care of a pediatric endocrinologist.

KEY POINTS

- DKA may present with tachypnea as the only recognizable sign or symptom.
- Never treat DKA with insulin boluses.
- If you must intubate, make sure the post-intubation respiratory rate matches the pre-intubation respiratory rate to prevent further acidosis.

- Patients with DKA must be monitored closely for GCS, changes in mentation, blood glucose changes, and electrolyte abnormalities.
- The safest place for pediatric patients in DKA to be managed is at pediatric facilities with experience in DKA management.

Further Reading

1. Chroboczek T, Cour M, Hernu R, Baudry T, et al. Long-term outcome of critically ill adult patients with acute epiglottitis. *PLoS One.* 2015;10(5):e0125736.
2. Isakson M, Hugosson S. Acute epiglottitis: epidemiology and Streptococcus pneumoniae serotype distribution in adults. *J Laryngol Otol.* 2011;125(4):390–393.
3. Stroud RH, Friedman NR. An update on inflammatory disorders of the pediatric airway: epiglottitis, croup, and tracheitis. *Am J Otolaryngol.* 2001;22(4):268–275.
4. Klingensmith GJ, Tamborlane WV, Wood J, Haller MJ, et al. Diabetic ketoacidosis at diabetes onset: still an all too common threat in youth. *J Pediatr.* 2013;162(2):330–334 e331.
5. Wolfsdorf JI, Glaser N, Agus M, Fritsch M, et al. ISPAD Clinical Practice Consensus Guidelines 2018: Diabetic ketoacidosis and the hyperglycemic hyperosmolar state. *Pediatr Diabetes.* 2018;19(Suppl 27):155–177.
6. Kuppermann N, Ghetti S, Schunk JE, Stoner MJ, et al. Clinical trial of fluid infusion rates for pediatric diabetic ketoacidosis. *N Engl J Med.* 2018;378(24):2275–2287.
7. Curtis JR, Bohn D, Daneman D. Use of hypertonic saline in the treatment of cerebral edema in diabetic ketoacidosis (DKA). *Pediatr Diabetes.* 2001;2(4):191–194.
8. Deeter KH, Roberts JS, Bradford H, Richards T, et al. Hypertension despite dehydration during severe pediatric diabetic ketoacidosis. *Pediatr Diabetes.* 2011;12(4 Pt 1):295–301.

17 He Went Wee, Wee, Wee All Night Long

Ajay K. Puri and Melissa A. McGuire

An overweight 15-year-old African American male with a history of developmental delay presents to your emergency department complaining of increased thirst, urinary frequency, nocturnal enuresis, decreased appetite and a 20-pound weight loss. His parents have type 2 diabetes. His temperature is 97.1°F, heart rate 126 bpm, blood pressure 114/85 mmHg, respiratory rate 20 breaths per minute, and oxygen saturation 96% on room air. A fingerstick glucose is obtained showing HI. Physical exam was notable for dry mucous membranes, tachycardia, and tachypnea without increased work of breathing. His initial complete blood count is significant for a white blood cell count of 15.85 K/uL, and a basic metabolic panel shows a sodium of 146 mmol/L, potassium of 5.2 mmol/L, chloride of 108 mmol/L, bicarbonate of 17 mmol/L, and glucose of 1216 mg/dL. A venous blood gas shows a pH of 7.27 and lactate of 3.9 mmol/L. A urinalysis showed large glucosuria and small ketones.

What do you do now?

DISCUSSION

While the treatment of diabeteic ketoacidosis (DKA) is familiar to most clinicians, hyperosmolar hyperglycemic syndrome (HHS) management in pediatric patients presents a unique challenge with a paucity of data to guide management. Patients in HHS are often treated with DKA protocols; however, they have important pathophysiologic differences that need to be reflected in planning a therapeutic approach.

EPIDEMIOLOGY

The incidence of both type 2 diabetes mellitus (T2DM) and HHS are increasing, with the majority of pediatric patients with T2DM obese or overweight. Two to 4% of children with T2DM will have HHS at initial presentation. T2DM patients who are male, obese, and African American are at highest risk for HHS. HHS in pediatrics carries a high mortality rate of 12% to 14%, making it an important clinical entity to be familiar with in emergency departments.

DIAGNOSIS

Initial investigations should include a fingerstick glucose, a basic metabolic panel, and venous blood gas to assess for acidosis and presence of an anion gap; testing of remaining electrolytes (magnesium, calcium, phosphorus) that are frequently deranged in this condition; a urinalysis to assess for ketonuria; a serum osmolality; and a creatine kinase to assess for rhabdomyolysis.

According to the American Diabetes Association and the International Society for Pediatric and Adolescent Diabetes, the criteria for diagnosis of HHS are as follows:

- Plasma glucose concentration > 600 mg/dL
- Venous pH >7.25; arterial pH >7.30
- Serum bicarbonate > 15 mmol/L
- Effective serum osmolality >320 mOsm/kg
- Small ketonuria, mild to absent ketonemia
- Altered consciousness or seizures

Patients presenting with HHS often face diagnostic delays. The severe hypertonicity in HHS leads to preservation of intravascular volume, making signs of dehydration potentially less obvious. Moreover, obesity can make the assessment of dehydration unreliable. In a case series by Price et al., three out of five cases had preceding health visits with nonspecific symptoms such as abdominal pain and headaches. Polyuria and polydipsia may be absent or not realized by the patient as the disease occurs indolently. A point-of-care blood glucose level should be considered in obese patients with nonspecific symptoms such as headache, weakness, abdominal pain, and vomiting. If severely dehydrated, patients with HHS can be acidotic from severe metabolic lactic acidosis.

It is important to note that DKA and HHS exist at the ends of a spectrum rather than as exclusive clinical entities and patients may present with features of both. This is discussed in greater detail later in this chapter.

INITIAL RESUSCITATION

1. Patients with HHS have approximately twice the total body fluid deficits compared to patients with DKA. Patients should be aggressively fluid resuscitated with 0.9% normal saline. Initiate a 20 ml/kg bolus and administer additional fluid boluses as required to restore peripheral perfusion.

2. Insulin administration is typically unnecessary early in classic HHS. Fluid administration and volume expansion causes a sharp decline in the glucose concentration. It is important to remember that glucose within the intravascular space exerts the osmotic pressure contributing to the maintenance of blood volume in this volume-depleted state. As such, a rapid decline in serum glucose concentration may cause circulatory collapse. Early insulin administration may accelerate circulatory dysfunction. However, insulin may be required in patients with severe ketosis and acidosis. Potassium deficits may also be worsened with insulin administration.

3. Once renal function is established, potassium replacement should be started for any patient whose serum potassium values are in the normal or low range: 40 mmol/L of potassium may be added

to replacement fluids and titrated up once an insulin infusion is started. The patient needs to be on a constant cardiac monitor. A summary of initial resuscitation and maintenance can be seen in Figure 17.1.

ONGOING RESUSCITATION

Fluid Resuscitation
After peripheral perfusion is established, 0.45% to 0.75% NaCl is used to replace the deficit over 24 to 48 hours with the goal of gradually correcting sodium. Urinary losses should be replaced.

Insulin Therapy
Insulin may be initiated when serum glucose is no longer declining at a rate of ~50 mg/dL per hour with fluid resuscitation alone. The initial infusion rate should be 0.025 to 0.05 U/kg/h and titrated to achieve a decrease in blood glucose of ~50 mg/dL/hr. The insulin infusion should be stopped once normoglycemia has been achieved if there is no concurrent acidosis.

Electrolytes
Deficits in potassium, magnesium, and phosphate are greater in HHS compared to DKA and require close monitoring.

Potassium replacement is usually required and serial values should be monitored every 2 to 3 hours. This may need to be done hourly if the patient is hypokalemic to ensure adequate repletion. For this reason, bicarbonate is contraindicated as it can exacerbate hypokalemia.

Phosphate deficiency may lead to multiple complications in HHS such as rhabdomyolysis. While administration is associated with an increased risk of hypocalcemia, an intravenous solution containing 50:50 of potassium chloride and potassium phosphate should sufficiently replete phosphate without driving hypocalcemia. Serum concentrations should be measured every 3 to 4 hours.

Magnesium serum levels should be obtained and monitored. The suggested dose is 25 to 50 mg/kg per dose for 3 to 4 doses every 4 to 6 hours at a maximum of 150 mg/kg/min or 2g/hr.

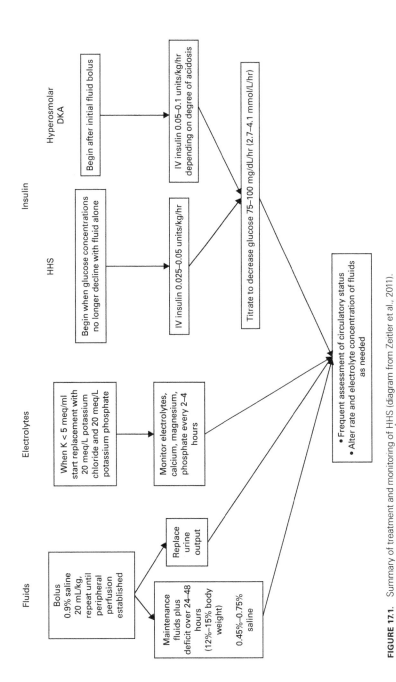

FIGURE 17.1. Summary of treatment and monitoring of HHS (diagram from Zeitler et al., 2011).

The degree of hypernatremia needs to be corrected in patients with HHS due to their high glucose levels in order to appreciate the severity and to obtain an accurate calculated serum osmolality. Hypernatremia should be corrected at a rate 0.5 mmol/L/hr.

COMPLICATIONS

Thrombosis

Thrombosis associated with central venous catheters (CVCs) is a common complication in HHS, for which heparin may be considered as prophylaxis. It is known that low-dose heparin may cause severe gastrointestinal bleeding due to hypertonicity-induced gastroparesis. Hence, heparin is recommended only in patients requiring CVCs for venous access or physiologic monitoring, or patients that are immobile for more than 24 to 48 hours.

Rhabdomyolysis

Rhabdomyolysis may occur in patients with HHS and lead to severe hyperkalemia, acute kidney injury, and hypocalcemia which may progress to cardiac arrest. Creatine kinase (CK) levels need to be obtained every 2 to 3 hours to assist with early detection. Since this process may lead to a potentially fatal complication, rising CK levels should prompt emergent nephrology consultation.

Malignant Hyperthermia

Multiple case reports describe signs and symptoms consistent with malignant hyperthermia in patients with HHS. Multiple causes have been suggested, the most popular being simple rhabdomyolysis, or as a reaction to a preservative in modern insulin formulations. The latter theory is supported by the fact that the syndrome often occurs after insulin administration. Nevertheless, a fever and rising CK levels may be treated with dantrolene.

Cerebral Edema

Altered mental status at presentation is common among patients in the hyperosmolar state and should improve with fluid resuscitation. Further investigation is warranted if patients continue to have declining mental status in spite of improving serum osmolality. Patients need to be monitored for headaches and changes in mental status. Electrolyte derangements, hypertonicity, and extreme dehydration are far more frequent causes of death than cerebral edema. Concerns about the possibility of causing cerebral edema should not dissuade adequate fluid resuscitation.

MIXED DKA AND HHS

Although DKA and HHS are distinct from one another in terms of diagnostic criteria, these can occasionally overlap. A patient with DKA may have severe osmolality, and HHS presents less frequently in the pediatric population compared to DKA, making recognition of HHS more difficult. Treatment of these "mixed" presentations needs to take into account possible complications of both. Treatment of HHS requires a higher rate of fluid administration compared to DKA, as fluid losses in HHS are doubled those of DKA. If insulin is required, hemodynamic status needs to be closely monitored, as insulin administration will lead to an increased rate of decline in serum glucose, possibly decreasing intravascular volume and perfusion. Guidelines to adjusting insulin and dextrose should mimic those in DKA with increased attention to monitoring of circulatory status and consequent adjustment to rates of fluid administration. Cerebral edema is more common in patients that present in mixed presentations, and hence monitoring of mental status is imperative. The goal is to establish adequate circulatory volume and cerebral perfusion, keeping in mind these patients typically require more fluid than classic DKA patients, but to also avoid unnecessary fluid administration.

Patients with HHS or a mixed picture typically require admission to the intensive care unit for ongoing resuscitation and monitoring.

CONCLUSION/DIAGNOSIS: HYPEROSMOLAR HYPERGLYCEMIC SYNDROME

This patient had a measured serum osmolality of 403 mOsm/kg and corrected to 362 mOsm/kg. At this point, the patient was diagnosed with HHS.

An initial fluid bolus of 20 ml/kg 0.9% normal saline was given followed by a subsequent 10 ml/kg bolus before switching to 0.45% normal saline for maintenance and urinary replacement. His glucose was 979 and 773 after each bolus, respectively. Intravenous potassium replacement was started, and he was admitted to the pediatric intensive care unit. Laboratory values were obtained every 2 hours to ensure a gradual decrease in sodium levels and maintenance of potassium, calcium, phosphate, and magnesium levels. An insulin infusion was started at 0.03 U/kg/hr in consultation with endocrinology and continued until a blood glucose below 300 was reached, and he was consequently started on glargine and aspart insulin subcutaneously. He was tested for glutamic acid decarboxylase, insulin antibody, and islet cell antibody, all of which were negative.

He was discharged home in stable clinical condition on his fourth day of hospitalization, after educating him and his parents on his insulin regimen.

KEY POINTS

- A fingerstick blood glucose level should be obtained liberally in obese patients, particularly male and African American patients with nonspecific symptoms, to assess for possible HHS.
- Patients may present with both DKA and HHS, and a treatment plan needs to address possible complications of both.
- The hallmark of HHS is rapid fluid resuscitation; cerebral edema is a rare complication in contrast to complications of underresuscitating these patients.
- Insulin therapy should be withheld until adequate fluid resuscitation has been achieved.

- Close attention needs to be paid to electrolyte levels and avoiding thrombosis, rhabdomyolysis, and malignant hyperthermia.
- Cerebral edema should be suspected if a patient's mental status deteriorates with resuscitation instead of improving.

Further Reading
1. Wolfsdorf J, Glaser N, Agus M et al. ISPAD Clinical Practice Consensus Guidelines 2018: Diabetic ketoacidosis and the hyperglycemic hyperosmolar state. *Pediatr Diabetes*. 2018;19:155–177. doi:10.1111/pedi.12701
2. Zeitler P, Haqq A, Rosenbloom A, Glaser N. Hyperglycemic hyperosmolar syndrome in children: pathophysiological considerations and suggested guidelines for treatment. *J Pediatr*. 2011;158(1):9–14.e2. doi:10.1016/j.jpeds.2010.09.048
3. Cochran J, Walters S, Losek J. Pediatric hyperglycemic hyperosmolar syndrome: diagnostic difficulties and high mortality rate. *Am J Emerg Med*. 2006;24(3):297–301. doi:10.1016/j.ajem.2005.10.007
4. Price A, Losek J, Jackson B. Hyperglycaemic hyperosmolar syndrome in children: patient characteristics, diagnostic delays and associated complications. *J Paediatr Child Health*. 2015;52(1):80–84. doi:10.1111/jpc.12980
5. Bassham B, Estrada C, Abramo T. Hyperglycemic hyperosmolar syndrome in the pediatric patient. *Pediatr Emerg Care*. 2012;28(7):699–702. doi:10.1097/pec.0b013e31825d23c9

18 The Not-So-Happy Wheezer

Hannah Carter and Isabel Barata

A previously healthy 4-month-old male presents to the
emergency department (ED) with shortness of breath
for the last 10 hours. Mom has noticed rhinorrhea,
cough, decreased oral intake, and a low-grade fever that
has now progressed to fast breathing. He is up-to-date
with his vaccinations, has no smoking exposure, and
attends day care. Family history is negative for asthma.

Vital signs are: temperature 38.2°C, heart rate 150,
respiratory rate (RR) 75, and oxygen saturation 90%
on room air. The exam is notable for a tachypneic
infant with a slightly sunken anterior fontanel,
nasal flaring, bilateral coarse breath sounds with
inspiratory and expiratory wheezing, and increased
work of breathing (WOB) with moderate subcostal
and intercostal retractions. He is sleepy but makes eye
contact. The patient is given supplemental oxygen.
Two hours later, patient is still in the ED and working
hard to breathe on 2 L NC oxygen with an oxygen
saturation of 89%. Mother is anxious and asks if there
is anything else you can do.

What do you do now?

DIAGNOSIS

In a healthy infant presenting with difficulty breathing associated with a fever, increased WOB, and wheezing, consider bronchiolitis, pneumonia, and asthma. If the child has a history of a significant pre-existing disease such as congenital heart disease, cystic fibrosis, or prematurity, consider more complicated cardiopulmonary pathology or be prepared for a potentially more complicated course. Pneumonia is unlikely given the diffuse wheezing without a focal lung exam. Asthma is unlikely given no history of eczema, reactive airway disease, and the symptoms in the setting of rhinorrhea and fever. The patient in this case is otherwise healthy and likely suffers from bronchiolitis.

Bronchiolitis is a common viral infection of the lower respiratory tract that usually affects young infants under 2 years of age. A common presentation is rhinorrhea, increased WOB, and wheezing, which is caused by inflammation in the bronchioles of the lung. Laboratory studies, such as a complete blood cell count and complete metabolic profile, viral panel (RVP), or chest radiographs (CXR), are not helpful in diagnosis. Rather, history and physical is essential for diagnosis, treatment, and disposition of pediatric patients with bronchiolitis. Once the diagnosis of bronchiolitis is made, close attention to the changes in vital signs, day of illness, and hydration status must be taken into consideration when considering the child's disposition.

MANAGEMENT

Once the clinical diagnosis of bronchiolitis is made, stage the severity of the illness using the Bronchiolitis guidelines. These may be provided by your institution or can be referenced from, for example, the Children's Hospital of Philadelphia. Depending on the RR, WOB, mental status, oxygen requirement, suction requirement, breath sounds, and cough, each patient can be categorized into mild, moderate, or severe bronchiolitis (Table 18.1).

Our patient would be classified as severe bronchiolitis according to the guidelines. It would be appropriate to begin supportive care with (a) bulb suction, (b) antipyretics, and (c) hydration.[1,2] Nasal suctioning has been clinically proven to decrease hospital length of stay (LOS) in bronchiolitis.[3]

TABLE 18.1. **Baseline Assessment and Pathway Status Determination**

		Mild (0)	Moderate (1)	Severe (2)
RR	**<3 months**	30–60	61–80	>80
	3–<12 months	25–50	51–70	>70
	1y–2y	20–40	41–60	>60
WOB		None or mild	Intercostal retractions	Nasal flaring, grunting, head bobbing
Mental Status		Baseline	Fussy or anxious	Lethargic or inconsolable
Oxygen Requirement		None	<1.5 liters	>1.5 liters
Suctioning		Bulb	Wall/Bulb	Wall
Breath Sounds		Clear	Crackles, Wheezing	Diminished breath sounds or significant crackles, wheezing
Cough		Absent or mild	Moderate	Severe

Source. Children's Hospital of Philadelphia, ©2019. https://www.chop.edu/clinical-pathway/bronchiolitis-emergent-evaluation-and-treatment-clinical-pathway-initial. Reprinted with permission.

After/while providing supportive care, monitor patient vital signs with emphasis on RR and oxygen saturation.[4]

Respiratory Support: High-Flow Nasal Cannula or Nasal CPAP

After nasal suctioning, monitor the oxygen saturation (SpO2) and attempt to wean supplemental oxygen if possible while maintaining >90% SpO2. If the patient continues to require oxygen without improvement in RR and WOB, consider high-flow nasal cannula (HFNC) or nasal continuous positive airway pressure (nCPAP). Both modalities, HFNC and nCPAP, have been shown to be helpful in bronchiolitis patients.[5–16]

HFNC is administered at 2 L/kg/min[17] to provide positive pressure of 2 to 5 cm H2O. According to a randomized controlled study (RCT) in 2017,

HFNC did not reduce time on oxygen compared to standard therapy but reduced intensive care unit (ICU) stay.[15] Another study by Bressan showed that HFNC improves oxygen saturation levels and decreases in end-tidal carbon dioxide and RR.[18] Moreover, a multicenter RCT in 2018 showed HFNC in bronchiolitis lowered rates of escalation of care compared to standard therapy. In this study, escalation of therapy was triggered when patients experienced persistent tachycardia, tachypnea, hypoxemia.[19] There are rare complications associated with HFNC use—including barotrauma[20]—but in general HFNC provides effective positive pressure, circumventing the need for intubation and shortening ICU stays.

CPAP is another modality to provide positive pressure in patients with bronchiolitis to improve respiratory status.[21] A retrospective cohort published in 2014 showed significant improvement with nCPAP use in length of ventilation, pediatric intensive care unit (PICU) LOS, and hospital length of stay (LOS) in patients with bronchiolitis.[22] A 2019 Cochrane Database review covered multiple RCTs that showed that RR decreased in bronchiolitis on nCPAP. The review also was not able to find significant benefit in CPAP in decreasing intubation rates or ICU LOS.[23] Another systemic review of RCTs concluded that there is no evidence that CPAP reduces need for intubation.[24]

Comparing the literature on HFNC and CPAP, HFNC has better evidence of decreasing PICU LOS and intubation rates, while evidence on CPAP is less clear. There have also been studies to directly compare both modalities. A RCT published in 2017 found noninferiority of HFNC compared to nCPAP when evaluating for alternative respiratory support, intubation rate, duration of ventilation, and length of PICU stay.[8] Moreover, a retrospective study also found that there was no significant difference between HFNC and nCPAP in LOS in PICU, measure of partial pressure of carbon dioxide and pH, heart rate, RR, fraction of inspired oxygen, and SpO2 in management of bronchiolitis.[13]

In summary, starting HFNC on our patient would be most appropriate since there is data that HFNC decreases PICU admissions and intubation rates. CPAP is also an option, but more research is warranted in terms of secondary clinical endpoints. CPAP has also not been shown to be superior in outcomes when compared directly to HFNC.

After patient has been on the HFNC, monitor for any changes in vital signs including RR, oxygen saturation, and WOB. If the patient develops hemodynamic instability or apnea at any point, endotracheal intubation will be necessary. See Figure 18.1 for an approach summary.

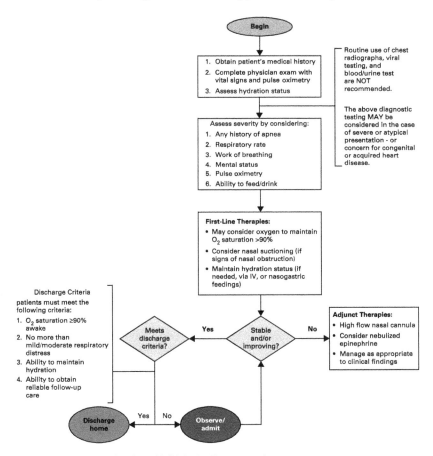

FIGURE 18.1. Approach to bronchiolitis in the Emergency department.
Adapted from "Clinical algorithm for Bronchiolitis in the Emergency Department Setting" publication by American Academy of Pediatrics' (AAP) Section on Emergency Medicine Committee on Quality Transformation (Ralston S et al. Pediatrics (2014) PMID 26430140)
**Assess severity: RR, WOB, Mental status, O2 requirement, suctioning, breath sounds, cough.
**First line tx: bulb suction, antipyretics, hydration
**Adjunct tx: HFNC, +/- CPAP

Also, it is important to recognize that the previously accepted treatments—albuterol,[25–29] steroids,[1] hypertonic saline,[30] antibiotics,[31] chest physiotherapy,[32] Heliox,[33] and leukotriene inhibitors[34]—have been proven through numerous studies to not provide treatment benefit in bronchiolitis.

DISPOSITION

The disposition of infants with bronchiolitis depends on the severity of their illness at presentation, their response to treatment, and their expected course of disease. If the patient improves with supportive care and continues to maintain SpO_2 >90%[1,4] at room air without signs of respiratory distress, consider discharge. Discuss the expected disease course and return precautions with parents; the patient can then be discharged with follow-up with a pediatrician in 1 to 2 days. Studies have shown that for mild/moderate cases of bronchiolitis, if patients are able to maintain oxygen saturation of 90% with appropriate WOB, RR with adequate oral intake, and reliable follow-up, they can be discharged.[35,36] In moderate to severe cases of bronchiolitis, care should be taken to monitor patients' vitals and respiratory status closely with each treatment. If they do not meet discharge criteria and they continue to require oxygen, they should be admitted. If a child requires HFNC, nCPAP, or intubation, he or she should be monitored in the ICU. Apnea or severe distress without improvement in the emergency room should also prompt an ICU admission.[35,36]

Also consider day of disease when deliberating admission. Lower respiratory symptoms peak in intensity during day 3 through 5.[37] Therefore, if patients present earlier than day 3, monitor closely for increased respiratory support and have a lower threshold for admission than a patient presenting on day 5.

KEY POINTS

- Consider bronchiolitis, pneumonia, and asthma in an infant with difficulty breathing.
- For an infant with a classic presentation of bronchiolitis, no diagnostic studies are indicated (including CXR, RVP, blood work).

- Bronchiolitis management is supportive with nasal suction, hydration, and fever control.
- HFNC is indicated for patients with moderate to severe bronchiolitis who require airway support (evidence supports decreased intubation rates and decreased PICU LOS). Evidence with CPAP is less clear.

Further Reading

1. Ralston SL, Lieberthal AS, Meissner HC, et al. Clinical practice guideline: the diagnosis, management, and prevention of bronchiolitis. *Pediatrics*. 2014;134:e1474.
2. Khoshoo V, Edell D. Previously healthy infants may have increased risk of aspiration during respiratory syncytial viral bronchiolitis. *Pediatrics*. 1999;104:1389.
3. Mussman GM, Parker MW, Statile A, et al. Suctioning and length of stay in infants hospitalized with bronchiolitis. *JAMA Pediatr*. 2013;167:414.
4. Wainwright CE, Kapur N. Oxygen saturation targets in infants with bronchiolitis. *Lancet*. 2015;386:1016.
5. Sinha IP, McBride AK, Smith R, Fernandes RM. CPAP and high-flow nasal cannula oxygen in bronchiolitis. *Chest*. 2015;148:810.
6. Pierce HC, Mansbach JM, Fisher ES, et al. Variability of intensive care management for children with bronchiolitis. *Hosp Pediatr*. 2015;5:175.
7. Wing R, James C, Maranda LS, Armsby CC. Use of high-flow nasal cannula support in the emergency department reduces the need for intubation in pediatric acute respiratory insufficiency. *Pediatr Emerg Care*. 2012;28:1117.
8. Milési C, Essouri S, Pouyau R, et al. High flow nasal cannula (HFNC) versus nasal continuous positive airway pressure (nCPAP) for the initial respiratory management of acute viral bronchiolitis in young infants: a multicenter randomized controlled trial (TRAMONTANE study). *Intensive Care Med*. 2017;43:209.
9. Franklin D, Babl FE, Schlapbach LJ, et al. A randomized trial of high-flow oxygen therapy in infants with bronchiolitis. *N Engl J Med*. 2018;378:1121.
10. McKiernan C, Chua LC, Visintainer PF, Allen H. High flow nasal cannulae therapy in infants with bronchiolitis. *J Pediatr*. 2010;156:634.
11. Schibler A, Pham TM, Dunster KR, et al. Reduced intubation rates for infants after introduction of high-flow nasal prong oxygen delivery. *Intensive Care Med*. 2011;37:847.
12. Kallappa C, Hufton M, Millen G, Ninan TK. Use of high flow nasal cannula oxygen (HFNCO) in infants with bronchiolitis on a paediatric ward: a 3-year experience. *Arch Dis Child*. 2014;99:790.

13. Metge P, Grimaldi C, Hassid S, et al. Comparison of a high-flow humidified nasal cannula to nasal continuous positive airway pressure in children with acute bronchiolitis: experience in a pediatric intensive care unit. *Eur J Pediatr.* 2014;173:953.
14. Mayfield S, Bogossian F, O'Malley L, Schibler A. High-flow nasal cannula oxygen therapy for infants with bronchiolitis: pilot study. *J Paediatr Child Health.* 2014;50:373.
15. Kepreotes E, Whitehead B, Attia J, et al. High-flow warm humidified oxygen versus standard low-flow nasal cannula oxygen for moderate bronchiolitis (HFWHO RCT): an open, phase 4, randomised controlled trial. *Lancet.* 2017;389:930.
16. Ganu SS, Gautam A, Wilkins B, Egan J. Increase in use of non-invasive ventilation for infants with severe bronchiolitis is associated with decline in intubation rates over a decade. *Intensive Care Med.* 2012;38:1177.
17. Milési C, Baleine J, Matecki S, et al. Is treatment with a high flow nasal cannula effective in acute viral bronchiolitis? A physiologic study. *Intensive Care Med.* 2013;39(6):1088–1094.
18. Bressan S, Balzani M, Krauss B, Pettenazzo A, Zanconato S, Baraldi E. High-flow nasal cannula oxygen for bronchiolitis in a pediatric ward: a pilot study. *Eur J Pediatr.* 2013;172(12):1649–1656.
19. Franklin D, Babl FE, Schlapbach LJ, et al. A randomized trial of high-flow oxygen therapy in infants with bronchiolitis. *N Engl J Med.* 2018;378(12):1121–1131.
20. Wing R, Armsby CC. Noninvasive ventilation in pediatric acute respiratory illness. *Clin Pediatr Emerg Med.* 2015;16:154–161.
21. Schuh S. Update on management of bronchiolitis. *Curr Opin Pediatr.* 2011;23:110.
22. Essouri S, Laurent M, Chevret L, et al. Improved clinical and economic outcomes in severe bronchiolitis with pre-emptive nCPAP ventilatory strategy. *Intensive Care Med.* 2014;40(1):84–91.
23. Jat KR, Mathew JL. Continuous positive airway pressure (CPAP) for acute bronchiolitis in children. *Cochrane Database Syst Rev.* 2019;1:CD010473.
24. Donlan M, Fontela PS, Puligandla PS. Use of continuous positive airway pressure (CPAP) in acute viral bronchiolitis: a systematic review. *Pediatr Pulmonol.* 2011;46:736.
25. Hartling L, Bialy LM, Vandermeer B, et al. Epinephrine for bronchiolitis. *Cochrane Database Syst Rev.* 2011;6:CD003123.
26. Skjerven HO, Hunderi JO, Brügmann-Pieper SK, et al. Racemic adrenaline and inhalation strategies in acute bronchiolitis. *N Engl J Med.* 2013;368:2286.
27. Gadomski AM, Scribani MB. Bronchodilators for bronchiolitis. *Cochrane Database Syst Rev.* 2014;6:CD001266.
28. Patel H, Gouin S, Platt RW. Randomized, double-blind, placebo-controlled trial of oral albuterol in infants with mild-to-moderate acute viral bronchiolitis. *J Pediatr.* 2003;142:509.

29. Cengizlier R, Saraçlar Y, Adalioğlu G, Tuncer A. Effect of oral and inhaled salbutamol in infants with bronchiolitis. *Acta Paediatr Jpn.* 1997;39:61.

30. National Institute for Health and Care Excellence. Bronchiolitis: diagnosis and management of bronchiolitis in children. Clinical Guideline NG 9. June 2015. https://www.nice.org.uk/guidance/ng9

31. Farley R, Spurling GK, Eriksson L, Del Mar CB. Antibiotics for bronchiolitis in children under two years of age. *Cochrane Database Syst Rev.* 2014;10:CD005189.

32. Roqué i Figuls M, Giné-Garriga M, Granados Rugeles C, Perrotta C. Chest physiotherapy for acute bronchiolitis in paediatric patients between 0 and 24 months old. *Cochrane Database Syst Rev.* 2012;2:CD004873.

33. Liet JM, Ducruet T, Gupta V, Cambonie G. Heliox inhalation therapy for bronchiolitis in infants. *Cochrane Database Syst Rev.* 2015;9:CD006915.

34. Liu F, Ouyang J, Sharma AN, et al. Leukotriene inhibitors for bronchiolitis in infants and young children. *Cochrane Database Syst Rev.* 2015;3:CD010636.

35. Scottish Intercollegiate Guidelines Network. Bronchiolitis in children. A national clinical guideline. 2006. www.sign.ac.uk/pdf/sign91.pdf

36. Bronchiolitis Guideline Team, Cincinnati Children's Hospital Medical Center. Bronchiolitis pediatric evidence-based care guidelines. 2010. www.cincinnatichildrens.org/service/j/anderson-center/evidence-based-care/recommendations/topic/

37. Thompson M, Vodicka TA, Blair PS, et al. Duration of symptoms of respiratory tract infections in children: systematic review. *BMJ.* 2013;347:f7027.

Sneezing, Wheezing, Having Trouble Breathing

Renee Quarrie

A 2-year-old girl with eczema is brought to the emergency department (ED) for shortness of breath. Three days ago she developed a dry cough and runny nose. The cough has progressively worsened and this morning her mother noted that she was short of breath. She has been well until this point except that she has wheezed 5 times before with colds and has needed "breathing treatments." She has never been admitted to the hospital. Her older sister and mother have asthma. She is not on any medications. Her mother says that she coughs a lot at night even when she is not sick. On examination she is sitting up in bed, tired appearing, and in obvious distress. She is afebrile, her heart rate is 148 per minute, respiratory rate is 48 per minute, oxygen saturation is 90%, and blood pressure is 98/62. She has subcostal, intercostal, and suprasternal retractions. On auscultation, air entry is significantly decreased throughout with inspiratory and expiratory wheezes. The remainder of her exam is normal.

What do you do now?

DISCUSSION

In a 2-year-old with no prior asthma diagnosis, the differential diagnosis for wheezing can be broad. The differential diagnosis includes (but is not limited to) asthma exacerbation, bronchiolitis (or other viral illness associated with wheezing), foreign body aspiration, esophageal foreign body, pneumonia, congenital structural causes, and cystic fibrosis. In this previously healthy patient, a diagnosis of cystic fibrosis is less likely and without a fever or focal lung findings, pneumonia is probably not the cause. Foreign body aspiration and esophageal foreign body usually lead to a more sudden onset of symptoms. Congenital structural causes usually present at a younger age and the symptoms are more consistent and persistent (especially with a fixed lesion). While this could certainly be a viral-induced wheezing given the prodrome of cough and runny nose, in this patient, an asthma exacerbation is the most likely diagnosis. There is key information in the history that makes an asthma exacerbation the most likely diagnosis. The patient has a history of atopy (eczema), has had prior wheezing episodes, and has a strong family history of asthma.

Asthma is one of the most common chronic diseases of childhood. The Global Initiative for Asthma defines it as follows: "Asthma is a heterogeneous disease, usually characterized by chronic airway inflammation. It is defined by the history of respiratory symptoms such as wheeze, shortness of breath, chest tightness, and cough that vary over time and in intensity, together with variable expiratory airflow limitation." The diagnosis of asthma using objective tests of airway obstruction (such as pulmonary function testing) is difficult in young children secondary to their inability to cooperate, therefore the diagnosis is largely clinical. The National Asthma Education and Prevention Program (NAEPP) recommends the modified Asthma Predictive Index as a tool for identifying children at increased risk for developing asthma (see Table 19.1).

A history of intermittent or chronic symptoms typical of asthma (see Table 19.2), plus the finding on physical examination of characteristic musical wheezing (present in association with symptoms and absent when symptoms resolve), strongly point to a diagnosis of asthma.

Diagnosis can be confirmed by spirometry if the child is old enough (around 5 years of age) to cooperate with testing. The evidence of airway

TABLE 19.1. **Modified Asthma Predictive Index**

Primary
≥ 4 wheezing episodes

AND	At least one major or two minor criteria	
Secondary	**Major Criteria**	**Minor Criteria**
	Parental history of asthma	Wheezing unrelated to colds
	Physician diagnosed atopic dermatitis	Eosinophils ≥ 4% in circulation
	Allergic sensitization to at least one aeroallergen	Allergic sensitization to milk, eggs, or nuts

obstruction on spirometry, especially if it can be reversed with a bronchodilator, is highly supportive of an asthma diagnosis. Measurements should include the forced vital capacity (FVC) and the forced expiratory volume in one second (FEV1). Airflow obstruction is defined as a FEV1 of 80%, or less than the expected volume for a healthy child, and a FEV1/FVC ratio of less than 85%. There are reference tables based on age, sex, race and height. The FEV1/FVC ratio appears to be a more sensitive measure of impairment than FEV1, whereas FEV1 may be a more useful measure of risk for future exacerbations. Spirometry should be performed before and after administration of a bronchodilator to assess for reversibility, with the established threshold being an increase of at least 9% in the FEV1.

This patient is presenting to the ED with an acute asthma exacerbation and needs immediate treatment. There are several ordinal scales used for the assessment of the initial severity of the asthma exacerbation. For

TABLE 19.2. **Symptoms of Asthma**

Cough—dry and hacking, usually worse at night	Chest tightness, pain, or pressure
Shortness of breath	Symptoms that are worse in certain pollen seasons (e.g., trees in early spring)
Wheezing	Concurrent flaring of other allergic symptoms such as rhinitis and eczema

this discussion the Pediatric Respiratory Assessment Model (PRAM) (Table 19.3) is used, but other ordinal scales such as the Pulmonary Index Score, Pediatric Asthma Severity Score, and the RAD score (Respiratory rate, Accessory muscle use, and Decreased breath sounds) have also been validated repeatedly in their assessment of asthma exacerbation severity. The goals of therapy in this patient should be rapid reversal of her airflow obstruction, correction of her hypoxemia, and reduction in likelihood of recurrence. By the PRAM criteria she is having a moderate asthma exacerbation.

TABLE 19.3. **Pediatric Respiratory Assessment Measure (PRAM)**

Score	Scalene muscle contraction	Suprasternal retractions	Wheezing	Air entry	Oxygen saturation on room air
0			Absent	Normal	>93%
1			Expiratory only	Decreased at bases	90%–93%
2	+	+	Inspiratory and Expiratory	Widespread decrease	<90%
3			Audible without stethoscope/ Silent chest with minimal air entry	Absent	

PRAM Clinical Score	Severity classification
0–4	Mild
5–8	Moderate
9–12	Severe
12 and lethargy, cyanosis, carbon dioxide retention, decreasing respiratory effort	Impending respiratory failure

Adapted from Chalut DS, Ducharme FM, Davis GM. The Preschool Respiratory Assessment Measure (PRAM): a responsive index of acute asthma severity. *J Pediatr.* 2000;137:762.

Supportive care includes administration of supplemental oxygen and fluids as necessary with very close monitoring of these patients and their response to therapy. Arterial blood gas analysis is only rarely needed in children with an acute asthma exacerbation as oxygen saturation can be assessed with pulse oximetry and, in severe asthma exacerbations, measurement of $PaCO_2$ may be obtained by noninvasive end-tidal CO_2 monitoring or capillary/venous blood gas samples. Studies have shown capillary blood gas and venous blood gas pCO_2 correlate significantly with arterial blood gas pCO_2, making them useful alternatives. End-tidal CO_2 monitoring also has been shown to correlate with arterial CO_2 as an effective noninvasive monitoring tool. Likewise, chest radiographs do not typically provide information that will alter the management of these patients and so they should only be performed in the presence of focal lung findings such as crackles, fever, or severe disease or in cases where there is uncertainty about the diagnosis.

In the patient with a mild asthma exacerbation, standard treatment begins with a dose of an inhaled beta-agonist, such as albuterol. Albuterol is the most commonly used bronchodilator. Levalbuterol is an active isomer of albuterol; it is often used in children who have a significant tachycardic response to albuterol, but it has not been shown to be more effective than albuterol and is more expensive, as such, it is rarely used as the first line of treatment in the ED. Clinical trials and meta-analyses indicate that the administration of beta-agonists via metered dose inhalers (MDIs) is at least as effective and possibly superior to the delivery of medication by nebulization in reversing bronchospasm in infants and children. However, it must be ensured that parents and patients are taught how to use MDIs correctly, and they should always use a spacer to ensure proper delivery of medication. Data suggests that 4 to 6 puffs of albuterol via MDI and spacer is equivalent to 2.5 mg of albuterol by nebulizer. Patients using a MDI with spacer may experience fewer side effects such as vomiting, tremors, hypoxemia, and tachycardia as compared with those using a nebulizer. Nebulized treatments are advantageous in some instances due to the ability to deliver humidified oxygen, and other medications, such as ipratropium bromide simultaneously with albuterol and drug therapy, can be passively administered to a child in respiratory distress. In addition, systemic steroids (usually oral) are administered as early as possible. Their effect is typically noted within 2 to

4 hours of administration. Their anti-inflammatory properties reduce the airway edema and secretions seen during asthma exacerbations.

In patients with moderate and severe exacerbations, many will have hypoxemia as a result of ventilation/perfusion mismatch, and if the oxygen saturation is less than 92%, the patient should be placed on supplemental oxygen. Beta-agonists may worsen this mismatch by causing pulmonary vasodilation in areas of the lung that are not well ventilated, and therefore nebulized medications should also be delivered with oxygen in these patients. Albuterol (see Table 19.4 for dosing) should be administered every 20 minutes intermittently for 3 doses or the 3 doses can be delivered continuously in the first hour.

Ipratropium bromide is an anticholinergic agent that causes smooth muscle relaxation and consequently bronchodilation. It is typically administered with the first three albuterol treatments and has been shown to reduce hospital admissions and improve lung function in children with severe asthma exacerbations. It has not been shown to reduce the length of hospital stay or prevent intensive care admission and, as such, only 3 doses need to be given during the acute management. Systemic corticosteroids are administered as early as possible in a moderate to severe asthma exacerbation, as early administration of steroids is associated with reduced admission rates. The NAEPP guidelines endorse a preference of oral administration of steroids (if possible) over intravenous administration as it is less invasive and has equivalent effect. Prednisone/prednisolone and dexamethasone are the corticosteroids typically used orally in the ED (see Table 19.4 for dosing). In severely ill patients, intravenous access should be established early and intravenous methylprednisolone can be administered if the patient is unable to take the corticosteroid orally.

If there is no significant clinical improvement or if the patient deteriorates despite treatment, in addition to continuous albuterol, intravenous magnesium sulfate can be administered. Because magnesium sulfate causes smooth muscle relaxation, a rare but important side effect of its infusion is clinically significant hypotension. To mitigate this, a normal saline bolus can be administered prior to or during the infusion. At a minimum, monitor the child's blood pressure closely with administration.

TABLE 19.4. **Doses of Medications Recommended to Treat Children During an Acute Asthma Exacerbation**

Medication	Dose
Albuterol by nebulizer	0.15 mg/kg/dose (minimum 2.5 mg, maximum 5 mg/dose) every 2 minutes for 3 doses Then 0.15–0.3 mg/kg (maximum 10 mg) every 30 minutes—4 hours as needed or switch to continuous therapy. Continuous Albuterol: 0.5 mg/kg/hour (maximum 20 mg/hour)
Ipratropium bromide by nebulizer	<20kg—250 mcg/dose ≥20kg—500 mcg/dose Every 20 to 30 minutes for 3 doses
Prednisone/ Prednisolone	1–2 mg/kg (once daily or divided twice a day); maximum 60 mg/day Oral 3–10 day course
Dexamethasone	0.6 mg/kg; maximum 16 mg/day Oral/IM/IV Single dose or once daily for 2 days
Methylprednisolone	1–2 mg/kg; maximum 125 mg/day IV
Magnesium Sulfate	25–75 mg/kg/dose; maximum 2.5 grams IV Infuse over 20 minutes
Epinephrine	0.01 mg/kg IM/SC; maximum 0.4 mg/dose May be repeated every 10–20 minutes for 3 doses
Terbutaline	0.01 mg/kg IM/SC; maximum 0.25 mg/dose May be repeated every 20 minutes for 3 doses then every 2–6 hours as needed Continuous infusion: 10 mcg/kg bolus over 10 minutes then 0.3–0.5 mcg/kg/minute infusion titrated to a max of 5 mcg/kg/minute

Note. IV = intravenous; IM = intramuscular; SC = subcutaneous; mcg = microgram.

For children with severe exacerbations not responding to therapy or in those with poor inspiratory flow who cannot cooperate with nebulizer treatment, intramuscular or subcutaneous epinephrine or terbutaline can be administered (see Table 19.4 for dosing). A continuous infusion of terbutaline can also be started if there is no improvement after magnesium sulfate infusion and continuous albuterol.

If the patient is not responding to the treatment regimens outlined here and is in significant distress, it is reasonable to consider noninvasive positive pressure ventilation (NPPV), such as bilevel positive airway pressure or continuous positive airway pressure. These are increasingly used to treat severely ill children due to the theoretical benefit of decreasing the effort of already fatigued respiratory muscles and preventing airway collapse upon exhalation. Contraindications to noninvasive techniques include altered mental status, hemodynamic instability, and multisystem organ failure.

If the child develops respiratory failure, endotracheal intubation is necessary. Intubation should be approached with caution in these patients, however, as their airways are already hyperresponsive and manipulation can lead to increased obstruction. Unfortunately, acute decompensation after intubation can also occur, so the healthcare team should be prepared. Indications for intubation in the patient with an acute exacerbation include hypoxemia despite high concentrations of oxygen or NPPV, severe increased work of breathing, altered mental status, and respiratory or cardiac arrest. Hypercarbia by itself is not an indication for intubation, but if there is a rapidly rising arterial partial pressure of carbon dioxide causing respiratory acidosis and altered mental status despite maximal therapy and NPPV, then the patient should be prepared for intubation. When choosing an agent for sedation, ketamine is the drug of choice due to its bronchodilatory properties.

Disposition of the wheezing patient is based on clinical and social factors. The patient who has marked improvement in clinical status (resolved or markedly improved wheezing, resolution of respiratory distress, increased aeration) within the first hour or two of treatment can be discharged home. It is important to note that while a peak flow meter may be used to assess airflow obstruction and provide an objective assessment of disease severity, it is rarely used during an acute exacerbation. The patient should have a beta-agonist available for use at home and should be educated on its use. A beta-agonist should be administered every 4 hours for the first 1 to 3 days after the ED visit and then every 4 hours as needed. The patient needs to be continued on prednisone or prednisolone following his or her first dose in the ED, and the course should be continued for up to 10 days (3–5 days should suffice in most patients). There is no need to taper steroid doses if administered for less than 10 days. If the patient received dexamethasone, the provider can choose to continue the medication for another day if clinically indicated.

Children who were severely ill upon presentation or who have little or insufficient improvement after initial therapy should be admitted to the hospital for continued management. Other criteria for admission include hypoxia, altered mental status, poor adherence with outpatient medication regimen, requiring beta-agonist therapy more frequently than every 4 hours, and inadequate access to emergency medical care.

Early recognition and intervention are critical for successful management of asthma exacerbations. The basic principles of management in these patients are assessment of severity, inhaled beta-agonists, early corticosteroid administration, supplemental therapy as needed, and frequent reassessment to determine response to therapy and escalate care as needed.

The patient in the scenario received 3 aerosols (combined albuterol/ipratropium) with moderate improvement. The patient was given an oral dose of prednisone prior to the first aerosol. After the aerosols the patient was watched for 2 hours with a return to a normal respiratory status and a pulse ox of 95%. The patient was discharged home to follow-up with her pediatrician.

KEY POINTS

- Asthma diagnosis in the pediatric patient is largely clinical. In patients with repeated wheezing and suggestive history, treat as an asthma exacerbation.
- Early recognition and intervention are critical for successful management of asthma exacerbations.
- Early administration of corticosteroids is important as it has been shown to reduce the rate of hospitalization.
- Routine chest radiographs do not play a part in the management of asthma.

Further Reading

Chalut DS, Ducharme FM, Davis GM. The Preschool Respiratory Assessment Measure (PRAM): a responsive index of acute asthma severity. *J Pediatr.* 2000;137:762.

Cronin JJ, McCoy S, Kennedy U, et al. A randomized trial of single-dose oral dexamethasone versus multidose prednisolone for acute exacerbations of asthma in children who attend the emergency department. *Ann Emerg Med.* 2016;67:593.

Global Initiative for Asthma. Global strategy for asthma management and prevention Updated 2015. http://www.ginasthma.org/local/uploads/files/GINA_Report_2015_Aug11.pdf

Griffiths B, Kew KM. Intravenous magnesium sulfate for treating children with acute asthma in the emergency department. *Cochrane Database Syst Rev.* 2016;4:CD011050.

National Asthma Education and Prevention Program: Expert panel report III: Guidelines for the diagnosis and management of asthma. (NIH publication no. 08-4051). Bethesda, MD: National Heart, Lung, and Blood Institute; 2007. www.nhlbi.nih.gov/guidelines/asthma/asthgdln.htm

Pardue Jones B, Fleming GM, Otillio JK, Asokan I, Arnold DH. Pediatric acute asthma exacerbations: evaluation and management from emergency department to intensive care unit. *J Asthma.* 2016 Aug;53(6):607–617.

Stenson EK, Tchou MJ, Wheeler DS. Management of acute asthma exacerbations. *Curr Opin Pediatr.* 2017 Jun 29;3:305–310.

20 Is There Anything Ultrasound Isn't Good For?

Trupti Shah and Athena Mihailos

A previously healthy 20-month-old female presents with abdominal pain, nausea, non-bilious, non-bloody vomiting, and lethargy for two days. Vital signs are: Temp: 99.6°F, BP: 86/58 mm/Hg, HR: 132 bpm, RR: 16 bpm, O_2 sat: 100%, and FS: 90. The physical exam was significant for a child lying very still with the legs flexed, tenderness to the right lower quadrant with involuntary guarding, and negative psoas and obturator signs. Intravenous fluids were initiated, nothing-by-mouth status was placed, presurgical labs were drawn, and pain control was provided.

What do you do now?

DISCUSSION

The answer is: a bedside ultrasound.

The differential of possible surgical emergencies that can be diagnosed via ultrasound for this patient's presentation includes appendicitis, intussusception, and ovarian torsion. The following is a discussion of each of these abdominal emergencies with their ultrasound findings.

INTRODUCTION

Abdominal pain is a common complaint of the pediatric population (age less than <18 years). It is the fourth most prevalent symptom in pediatric emergency department (ED) visits and sick office visits, accounting for 5% to 10% of all ED visits (1). It is a challenging complaint to assess; there is significant difficulty in drawing out associated symptoms, localizing the pain, and examining the abdomen in a small child. A large differential exists for the underlying cause of abdominal pain in children. This ranges from benign self-limited conditions such as gastroenteritis and constipation to more acute disease processes requiring surgical intervention such as ovarian torsion and appendicitis.

Ultrasound is accessible at the bedside, lacks radiation exposure to the patient, and has become a preferred initial method of imaging for pediatric patients in many acute scenarios. It has been embraced due to its accessibility; its rate of use has increased due to expanded interest in point of care ultrasound (POCUS).

ACUTE APPENDICITIS

Appendicitis is the most common surgical diagnosis for pediatric abdominal pain. Early recognition is paramount, especially with the trend toward nonsurgical management. Imaging options include both ultrasound and computed tomography (CT). Although CT scan has great sensitivity, has high specificity, and is not user dependent, as ultrasound is, it has decreased in popularity due to its increased risk of cancer secondary to radiation exposure, especially in children. Ultrasound has emerged as the initial imaging modality for acute appendicitis secondary to its decreased cost, increased availability, and use of non-ionizing radiation. The ability to perform an abdominal ultrasound to identify an appendix should be in every ED physician's arsenal.

Acute appendicitis should be considered in any child with abdominal pain with or without other additional clinical features including but not limited to right lower quadrant abdominal pain, migration of pain, nausea, vomiting, anorexia, rebound tenderness, pyrexia, or elevated white blood cell count (2). POCUS for appendicitis has been taught to emergency physicians with good reliability.

This particular scan should be performed with a linear high frequency transducer. Ideally, the patient should be NPO with a full bladder. A graded compression study (application of gentle pressure on the transducer to displace and compress any bowel loops underneath) would be performed with the patient in a supine position. Scanning is performed in two planes (sagittal and transverse) to identify the relevant structures. The iliac vessels and right psoas muscle should be located. The ascending colon should be followed inferiorly to identify the cecum and the appendix arising from it (Figure 20.1).

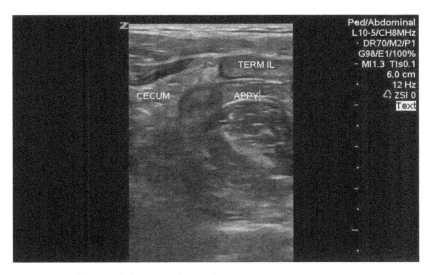

FIGURE 20.1. Ultrasound of cecum and appendix.

The terminal ileum is separate and is compressible with peristalsis. The appendix should be visualized in its entirety and measure 6 mm or less in diameter. The wall of the appendix should be thin, measuring less than 3 mm. It should be empty except for gas or stool and compressible with no hypervascularity. These are the findings of a normal appendix on ultrasound.

Acute appendicitis would appear differently on ultrasound. It may have an enlarged diameter (greater than 6 mm) or a thickened wall (greater than 3 mm). Lack of compressibility (unless perforated) and increased vascularity are also signs of abnormality (Figure 20.2A). The appendix may take on a target-like appearance in cross-section (Figure 20.2B). This is caused by a fluid-filled hypoechoic center with a hyperechoic ring of mucosa surrounded by a hypoechoic muscular layer. An appendicolith will appear as a hyperechoic focus with posterior shadowing. There are other ultrasound findings that are less specific for appendicitis but helpful in establishing the diagnosis if noted. Free fluid in the right lower quadrant or a periappendiceal abscess may be seen as well as enlarged lymph nodes. The surrounding fat may appear hyperechoic as well as the thickened overlying peritoneum (2).

Frequently, the appendix will not be identified during a scan. Repeating the ultrasound a few hours later has shown to significantly increase the sensitivity (3).

Factors associated with failure to identify the appendix include operator skill level, location of the appendix, body habitus, and tolerance of pain. A retrocecal appendix, or one displaced due to long length or malrotation, will be difficult to visualize. Adequate pain relief is encouraged prior to beginning the ultrasound in order to limit abdominal guarding and facilitate a detailed and thorough exam.

Other diagnoses that can mimic appendicitis clinically or sonographically that are important to consider include terminal ileitis, omental infarction, mesenteric adenitis, and ovarian pathology.

INTUSSUSCEPTION

Another common pediatric abdominal emergency to be considered in this patient is intussusception. It is a process in which a small segment of intestine

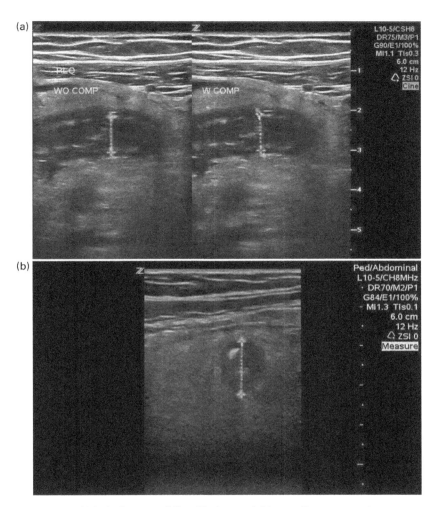

FIGURE 20.2. (a) Lack of compressibility with ultrasound. (b) target- like appearance in cross-section of appendix.

invaginates into an adjoining lumen, most frequently ileum into cecum. It is most common in the first 2 years of life and predominates in males. Most symptoms are very nonspecific, such as fussiness, nausea, vomiting, lethargy, and intermittent crampy abdominal pain. On physical exam the patient may have a "sausage-shaped" mass. Red currant jelly stools are a late finding denoting bowel ischemia (4). Ultrasound is the imaging modality of choice for its high sensitivity and specificity in experienced hands.

Abdominal ultrasonography for evaluating intussusception is performed in the patient in a supine position using a linear high resolution transducer. Usually, the sonographer begins in the right lower quadrant and sweeps the probe across the abdomen maintaining a cross-sectional view of the intestines. The patient's physical exam findings of a "sausage-shaped" mass may help direct the scan.

There a few common findings on ultrasound with intussusception. A target sign or bull's-eye sign is commonly seen in the transverse plane of the intussusception. It is created by the concentric alternating hyperechoic (mucosa and muscle) and hypoechoic (submucosa) bands of the layers of intestines (Figure 20.3A). This usually measures over 3 cm in diameter. A variation of this in which mesentery is pulled into the intussusception is known as "crescent in a doughnut" sign. In longitudinal view, an intussusception may appear to have a pseudokidney appearance (Figure 20.3B). The vessels of the fat containing mesentery can mimic a renal hilum and the edematous bowel has the appearance of renal parenchyma. If intussusception is suspected on ultrasound, it should be imaged in both planes. The possibility of spontaneous resolution of intussusception is something to be cognizant of and consider. Retrospective analyses have indicated that in the right clinical setting a highly suggestive abdominal radiograph with a mass, obstruction, or visible intussusception may be equivalent to ultrasound. This can substitute in cases where ultrasound is unattainable (5).

OVARIAN TORSION

Adnexal or ovarian torsion is rare in the pediatric population, accounting for approximately 3% of cases of abdominal pain. However, given the risk of complications from peritonitis, infection, sepsis, chronic pain, adhesions, and possible impact of future fertility, it is considered a surgical emergency. Ovarian torsion can occur at any age including neonatal period (16%) (6), so a high level of suspicion must be maintained in a population that may not be able to contribute to the history and clinical exam. The most common presenting complaint is usually acute onset of unilateral abdominal or pelvic pain of variable intensity, location, and duration. Previous

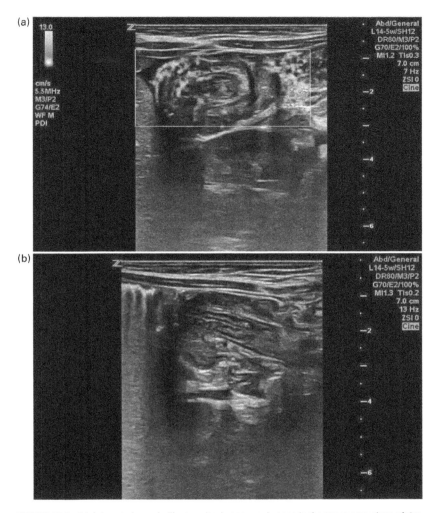

FIGURE 20.3 (a) A target sign or bull's-eye sign is commonly seen in the transverse plane of the intussusception. (b) In longitudinal view, an intussusception may appear to have a pseudokidney appearance

intermittent similar complaints should also raise clinical suspicion for this entity. Other supporting symptoms of nausea, vomiting, anorexia, and low-grade fever are nonspecific. Ultrasound is the most appropriate diagnostic imaging modality for this condition. Operator skill plays a substantial role in diagnostic accuracy (7).

In the pediatric population, a transabdominal approach to the pelvic ultrasound is usually attempted. It is imperative that the patient's pain is well controlled and the bladder is full in order to obtain the best images. This helps create an acoustic window for improved imaging. Normal adnexa for prepubertal to premenarchal girls range from 1 to 4 cm³. Postmenarche, there is an increase in size of the ovary to an average of 8 cm³. Normal follicle size prior to menarche is average 4 mm and total number less than 6.

There are a multitude of sonographic findings that can be associated with ovarian torsion in the pediatric population. The most common positive finding on ultrasound in cases of torsion is unilateral/asymmetric ovarian enlargement. The ovary is usually heterogeneous in appearance with edema. (Figure 20.4) A simple or complex adnexal mass or cyst may be seen. In a torsed ovary, absence of venous flow or both arterial and venous flow can be seen. This, along with free fluid surrounding the affected ovary or into Pouch of Douglas, were the most statistically significant findings for ovarian torsion (7).

A recent study showed that 2 or more positive findings on ultrasound increased the likelihood of the diagnosis significantly. Another study demonstrated that an ultrasound negative for torsion has a very high

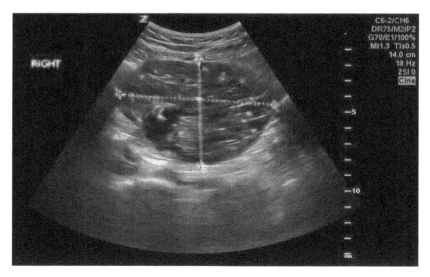

FIGURE 20.4 The ovary is usually heterogeneous in appearance with edema.

negative predictive value (8). In the adult population, the risk of ovarian torsion increases significantly when the ovary size is greater than 5 cm; however, children may frequently have torsion with normal sized ovaries (6).

Although ultrasound is very helpful in diagnosing ovarian torsion, it is still a clinical diagnosis and a surgical emergency. Definitive treatment is operative laparoscopy, with possible detorsion. In the past, an oophorectomy was reserved for cases of necrosis due to the potential for inflammation causing adhesions and possible small bowel obstruction (SBO) in the future. Recent data suggests that detorsion of a necrotic appearing ovary may preserve later function.

CONCLUSION

A POCUS study performed by the emergency medicine physician in the ED revealed a fluid-filled noncompressible tubular structure arising from the cecum on one end and blind-ended. The diameter measured 8 mm with a target like appearance and a small amount of free fluid surrounding it. A diagnosis of acute appendicitis was made, the patient was given antibiotics, and surgery was consulted to direct further management. The surgeon elected to remove the appendix, which was well tolerated. The patient remained in the hospital for one day and was discharged home with pain medication. Ultrasound was the modality that diagnosed this patient's appendicitis without exposing the infant to ionizing radiation, avoiding unnecessary sedation and providing a prompt and accurate diagnosis.

KEY POINTS

- Ultrasound has emerged as the initial imaging modality for acute appendicitis secondary to its decreased cost, increased availability, and use of non-ionizing radiation.
- Acute appendicitis on ultrasound may have an enlarged diameter (greater than 6 mm) or a thickened wall (greater than 3 mm). Lack of compressibility (unless perforated) and increased vascularity are also signs of abnormality.

· A target sign or bull's-eye sign is commonly seen in the transverse plane on ultrasound of intussusception.
· The most common positive finding on ultrasound in cases of torsion is unilateral/asymmetric ovarian enlargement.

Further Reading

1. Mittal, Manoj, et al. "Performance of Ultrasound and the Diagnosis of Appendicitis in Children in a Multicenter Cohort." *Academic Emergency Medicine*. 2013;20,7:697–702.
2. Quigley, Alan; Stafrace, Samuel. "Ultrasound Assessment of Acute Appendicitis in Pediatric Patients: Methodology and Pictorial Overview of Findings Seen." *Insights Imaging*. 2013;4:741–751.
3. Schuh, Suzanne, et al. "Properties of Serial Ultrasound Clinical Diagnostic Pathway in Suspected Appendicitis and Related Computed Tomography Use." *Academic Emergency Medicine*. 2015;22,4:406–414.
4. Riera, Antonio, et al. "Diagnosis of Intussusception by Physician Novice Sonographers in the Emergency Department." *Annals of Emergency Medicine*. 2012;60,3:264–268.
5. Mendez, Donna, et al. "The Diagnostic Accuracy of an Abdominal Radiograph with Signs and Symptoms of Intussusception." *American Journal of Emergency Medicine*. 2012;30:426–431.
6. Childress, Krista; Dietrich, Jennifer. "Pediatric Ovarian Torsion." *Surgical Clinics of North America*. 2017;97:209–221.
7. Mashiach, Reuven, et al. "Sonographic Diagnosis of Ovarian Torsion." *Journal of Ultrasound Medicine*. 2011;30:1205–1210.
8. Naiditch, Jessica; Barsness, Katherine. "The Positive and Negative Predictive Value of Transabdominal Color Doppler Ultrasound for Diagnosing Ovarian Torsion in Pediatric Patients." *Journal of Pediatric Surgery*. 2013;48:1283–1287.
9. Hernanz-Schulman, Marta, et al. "Hypertrophic Pyloric Stenosis in the Infant without Palpable Olive: Accuracy of Sonographic Diagnosis." *Pediatric Radiology*. 1994;193:771–776.
10. Sivitz, Adam, et al. "Evaluation of Hypertrophic Pyloric Stenosis by Pediatric Emergency Physician Sonography." *Academic Emergency Medicine*. 2013;20:646–651.
11. Dias, Silvia, et al. "Hypertrophic Pyloric Stenosis: Tips and Tricks for Ultrasound Diagnosis." *Insights Imaging*. 2012;3:247–250.

Index

electrolytes, 162–64

encephalitis, 135–36

encephalopathy, hypoxic-ischemic, 38

enemas, 106–7

Enterobacter, 14

Enterococcus, 14

enterocolitis

    food protein-induced, 89–90

    Hirschsprung-associated, 2, 4–5

enuresis, nocturnal, 159–67

epiglottitis, 150–51

epilepsy

    definition, 39–40

    recommended approach, 137, 138*t*

    syndromes, 39–40

epileptic seizures, 34

epinephrine, 185*t*, 186

Escherichia coli, 14

febrile seizures, 146–47

    complex, 135, 138*t*

    key points, 138–39

    simple, 135, 138*t*

febrile seizures simplex (FSs), 39–40

fever, 59–71

    case vignette, 59, 63–65

    in children 3 to 36 months, 65–66

    in children older than 3 years, 66

    high-risk criteria, 61–63, 63*t*

    in infants, 60–65, 64*t*, 67

    key points, 7–9, 67

    low-risk criteria, 15, 16*t*

    in neonates, 4–9, 13–22

    recommended empiric antibiotic therapy, 63, 64*t*

    risk stratification, 5–7

    step-by-step approach, 61–63, 63*t*, 67

    treatment, 4–5, 63, 64*t*, 67

    urine testing, 65–66

fifth day fits, 39–40

fluid-refractory shock, 79

fluids

    initial fluids in DKA, 153–54

    while on insulin, 154

food protein-induced enterocolitis, 89–90

formula, 89–90

fosphenytoin, 36–37, 37*t*, 38*t*, 132, 145

FSs (febrile seizures simplex), 39–40

fundoscopy, 124–25, 124*t*

gastroenteritis, 1, 7, 104

gastroesophageal reflux (GER), 84

gastroesophageal reflux disease (GERD), 84

gastrointestinal bugs, 111–21

gentamicin, 64*t*

GER (gastroesophageal reflux), 84

GERD (gastroesophageal reflux disease), 84

Glasgow Coma Score, 124–25, 124*t*

Group B Streptococcus, 14

Haddad syndrome, 3

HAEC (Hirschsprung-associated enterocolitis), 2, 4–5

HAEC score, 4–5, 6*t*

Haemophilus influenzae type b (Hib) vaccines, 60, 65, 135–36

happy spitters, 84

HD. *See* Hirschsprung's disease

headache, 123–29

    red flag symptoms warranting imaging consideration, 124–25, 124*t*

head trauma, 116

hematemesis (bloody vomiting), 84–89, 85*t*

herpes, 39

herpes simplex infections, 19

herpesvirus infection, 19

HFNC (high-flow nasal cannula), 171–74, 175

HHS. *See* hyperosmolar hyperglycemic syndrome

Hib (*Haemophilus influenzae* type b) vaccines, 60, 65, 135–36

HIE (hypoxic-ischemic encephalopathies), 38

high-flow nasal cannula (HFNC), 171–74, 175

diagnosis, 104, 105–6, 108
key points, 108
management, 106–7, 108
surgical small bowel intussusception
(SSBI), 108
ultrasound findings, 194, 195*f*
invasive bacterial infections (IBIs),
5–7, 14–15
ipratropium bromide, 184, 185*t*

ketamine, 146
Klebsiella, 14

Ladd's procedure, 119
Laurence-Moon-Biedl-Bardet syndrome, 3
leucovorin, 37*t*
levetiracetam, 36, 37*t*, 145
lidocaine, 36, 37*t*
lorazepam, 36, 37*t*, 132
lumbar puncture, 15–18, 18*f*, 127–28

magnesium replacement, 162
magnesium sulfate, 185*t*, 186
magnetic resonance imaging (MRI)
of brain, 125–26, 128
rapid, 125–26, 128
malignant hyperthermia, 164
Mallory-Weiss tear, 84–89
malrotation with volvulus, 118–19
case vignette, 111, 117–18
key points, 120
radiographic findings, 118*f*,
118–19, 120*f*
McBurney's point, 97
MDIs (metered dose inhalers), 184
meconium: failure to pass, 1–11
medications. *See also specific medications
by name*
for acute asthma exacerbation, 184,
185*t*, 188
antibiotics, 76–79, 77*f*, 98–99
anticonvulsants, 143–45
antiepileptic drugs (AEDs), 38, 145

for seizures, 36–37, 37*t*, 38*t*, 132,
141, 143–45
meningitis, 14, 135–36
mental status, altered, 124–25, 124*t*
metabolic acidosis, 151
metabolic disorders, 39
metered dose inhalers (MDIs), 184
methylprednisolone, 184, 185*t*
midazolam, 36–37, 37*t*, 38*t*, 132,
141, 143–45
midgut volvulus, 118–19
case vignette, 111, 117–18
double bubble sign, 117–19, 118*f*
key points, 120
whirl or whirlpool sign, 119–20, 120*f*
MRI. *See* magnetic resonance imaging
MUDPILES mnemonic, 152

nasal continuous positive airway pressure
(nCPAP), 171–74
NAT. *See* nonaccidental trauma
National Asthma Education and Prevention
Program (NAEPP), 180
necrotizing enterocolitis, 119
neglect, 115
neonatal hypoglycemia, 23–31, 39
case vignette, 23
causes, 26–28, 29*t*
definition, 24–25, 35–36
ED management, 35–36
epidemiology/incidence, 25
key points, 30
long-term sequelae, 30
pathophysiology, 25–26
persistent, 28, 29*t*
risk factors for, 27
screening and treatment, 28, 29*t*
signs and symptoms, 26, 27*t*
neonatal seizures, 33–43
benign idiopathic convulsions, 39–40
case vignette, 33, 42
common causes, 38–40
differential diagnosis, 132–34, 133*t*